Learning
for Children

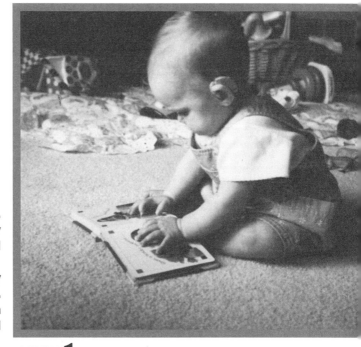

Lyn Robertson, Ph.D.
Denison University
Granville, OH

Introduction by
Carol Flexer, Ph.D.
University of Akron
Akron, OH

Who Are
Deaf or Hard
of Hearing

The Alexander Graham Bell Association for the Deaf and Hard of Hearing is
a membership organization and information clearinghouse on pediatric hearing loss, emphasizing the use of technology, speech, speechreading, residual
hearing, and written and spoken language. AG Bell focuses specifically on children with hearing loss, providing ongoing support and advocacy for parents,
professionals, and other interested parties.

AG Bell publishes books and brochures on the subject of hearing loss, auditory approaches in education, advocacy, employment, and advances in hearing
technology. AG Bell also publishes a magazine, *Volta Voices*, a scholarly journal,
The Volta Review, and offers resource/referral services to individuals with questions about hearing loss and auditory approaches.

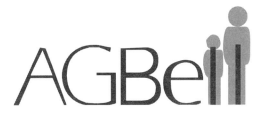

The Alexander Graham Bell Association for the Deaf
and Hard of Hearing
3417 Volta Place, N.W.
Washington, DC 20007-2778

Printed in the USA
10 9 8 7 6 5 4 3 2 1

Contents

Figures and Tables

Preface

M̲Y INTENTION IN WRITING THIS BOOK IS TO PRODUCE THE VOLUME I WOULD HAVE liked to have had in my hands 21 years ago when our daughter Annie was pronounced severe-to-profoundly deaf. I use the word "pronounced" because at the time it felt like a sentence laid on us, a terrible end to her wonderful babyhood. The audiologist who diagnosed her inability to hear warned us about three probabilities: (1) Annie would not be able to attend "regular" school until about fifth grade, if at all; (2) Annie probably wouldn't qualify for a college education and would probably end up doing menial work when she entered the job market; and (3) my husband and I could quite possibly end up divorcing. That audiologist was speaking from her experience with individuals who are deaf or hard of hearing. Each of her predictions really was quite likely from a statistical point of view, and we were devastated. And then we were determined somehow to do better than these predictions.

Fresh from my Master's degree studies in Reading and Language at Northwestern University, I knew enough to know that Annie was in real danger of not learning to speak, to read, and to write. From the first, my mother had a blind faith that once we put on the hearing aids ("plugged her in"), Annie would become part of the hearing world. Oddly enough, my mother was right, though it took us another year to find our way to people who were doing essentially that. Of course, there was more to it than just "plugging her in," but that was the place to start.

I am grateful to the many therapists who worked with Annie, to her teachers who took such care with her, and to all who took the time to talk with her so many years ago when communicating with her was hard — all of them together made it possible for her to learn to read and write by helping her build her own ability to use language.

As I write this, Annie has graduated from Kalamazoo College, a nationally known liberal arts college in Kalamazoo, Michigan, where she majored in Sociology and Anthropology, minored in writing, and completed a concentration in women's studies. She studied abroad in England and, after returning to campus, co-edited a publication on studying abroad. A little over a year ago, at age 21, she received a cochlear implant made necessary by a sudden, precipitous decline in the small amount of hearing she had. Because she was already accomplished at using her hearing, the implant allows her to hear more than any of us ever dreamed possible. Her first job after graduation is an admission counselor at Kalamazoo College. She also has been a co-editor of the college newspaper, a leader in a wilderness program for students, and an advisor to students in the Career Development Center.

None of her academic success could have happened if she had not learned to read, and so I want to pass on what I have learned about literacy and deafness to parents of newly diagnosed and/or implanted children, to therapists, and to teachers. Twenty years ago when we began our work with Annie, she wore a body-type hearing aid with a Y-cord and progressed to two ear-level hearing aids only because I persuaded a very kind audiologist/hearing aid dealer to fit her with them at age $2^1/_2$. She was the first child in our area that he had fitted that way. While we kept up with each new product that could help her hear better, Annie's first, critical years of hearing were not technologically sophisticated. So much more can be done today! My good friend Carol Flexer has graciously provided the Introduction describing how new amplification technologies are changing everything we used to "know" about deafness and being hard of hearing. And then, the title of each of my chapters is a question that you may be asking about literacy.

Also, I would like to thank the people of Natural Communication, Inc., in Northeast Ohio for providing me the photographs that are invaluable in illustrating many of the points made in this book.

I hope this book will be the guidance for you that I would like to have had before me during those early, uncertain years.

Lyn Robertson
June 16, 2000

How Are New Amplification Technologies Changing Everything That We Used to Know About Deafness?

Carol Flexer, Ph.D., Professor of Audiology
The University of Akron, Akron, Ohio

A S WE ENTER THE NEW MILLENNIUM, EVERYTHING WE THOUGHT WE KNEW ABOUT deafness has changed — dramatically. Why? New hearing aid and FM technology and cochlear implants have allowed access to critical auditory brain centers for stimulation of neural growth — brain centers that could not be accessed with previous and less effective generations of amplification technologies. Early identification has enabled us to fit amplification technology and cochlear implants on babies. Therefore, auditory language enrichment can be provided during critical periods of maximum brain neural plasticity — the first few years of life (Northern & Downs, 1991). As a result, today's babies and young children who are born deaf have incredible possibilities for achieving higher levels of spoken language, reading skills, and academic competencies than were available to most children in previous generations (Yoshinaga-Itano, 1998).

Recent census data show that while 82% of Americans, overall, complete high school (Manning, 1998), 43% of the students in special education programs do not (Boutte, 1998). Approximately 27% of the U.S. population has a bachelor's degree. People without a high school diploma earn an average of $15,011 a year; with a high school diploma, $22,154; with a bachelor's degree, $38,112; and with an advanced degree, $61,317 per year (Manning, 1998). The more education one has, the more pay one is likely to earn.

So what? After all, this book is about literacy learning for children who are deaf or hard of hearing, not about typically hearing children completing post-secondary education and obtaining adult employment. The fact is, the neuro-logical foundations we foster during the first critical years of a child's life — whether or not that child has a hearing loss — provide the "velcro" for the attachment of later linguistic, literary, and academic competencies (Gilbertson & Bramlett, 1998; Sharpe, 1994). It is possible, therefore, that in many instances when a child is unable to graduate from high school or to pursue post-secondary education, it is because we unintentionally diluted a powerful ingredient for brain integrity — audition. Or, as was the case in the past, many children who were born deaf or hard of hearing did not have an opportunity for auditory brain development because their hearing losses prevented audi-tory information from reaching the brain. No more!

Studies in brain development show that sensory stimulation of the auditory centers of the brain is critically important and, indeed, influences the actual organization of auditory brain pathways (Boothroyd, 1997; Chermak & Musiek, 1997; Musiek & Berge, 1998).

The same brain areas — the primary and secondary auditory areas — are most active when a child listens and when a child reads. That is, phonological or phonemic awareness, which is the explicit awareness of the speech SOUND structure of language units, forms the basis for the development of literacy skills (Gilbertson & Bramlett, 1998).

The point is, anything we can do to access and "program" those critical and pow-erful auditory centers of the brain with acoustic detail will expand children's oppor-tunities.

This Introduction will provide evidence that "hearing" is the most effective modality for the teaching of spoken language (speech), reading, and cognitive skills. Furthermore, with today's amplification technologies, cochlear implants and early identification and intervention, auditory brain access and develop-ment are available to babies with even the most profound deafness. Topics cov-ered include definitions and discussions of hearing loss, audiograms, amplifi-cation technologies, and listening skill development. In addition, auditory-verbal communication and intervention will be introduced. This Introduction concludes with a list of suggested readings about hearing, hearing loss, ampli-fication, and auditory-verbal practice.

Functional Definitions of the Terms "Hearing-Impaired," "Hard of Hearing," and "Deaf"

Three of the terms used most commonly to describe hearing loss are "hear-ing impairment," "hard of hearing," and "deaf." These terms can have various meanings, but in our opinion the definitions proposed by Mark Ross, an audiologist and a person who experiences a severe to profound hearing loss, are the most useful (Ross, Brackett, & Maxon, 1991). He uses "hearing impairment" to describe any type and degree of hearing loss. The terms "hard of hearing" and "deaf" are used *functionally*. These terms are not associated with time of onset of the hearing loss or with the audiometric degree of hearing loss. Rather, a person is *functionally hard of hearing* if he or she learned language primarily auditorally and if he or she receives information from the environment, primarily auditorally. So, a person could have been born with a profound hearing loss, but if amplification technology and auditory-verbal intervention enabled him or her to learn language primarily auditorally, then he or she would be functionally hard of hearing.

A person is *functionally deaf* if he or she learned language primarily visually and receives information from the environment primarily visually. Visual input includes lipreading, Cued Speech, and manual communication or sign language. Note that many traditional "oral" programs are as visually based in assumptions and teaching as are manual communication programs. Both assume that children with hearing impairments cannot use amplified auditory input as their *primary mode* for learning; they must focus on vision.

Mark Ross further elaborates on his proposed functional definitions by stating that a child or anyone with a hearing impairment who is functionally hard of hearing is much more like a typically hearing person relative to how information is learned than they are like someone who is functionally deaf. One who is functionally hard of hearing, through hearing aids or cochlear implants, accesses and develops the auditory centers of the brain in a similar manner as a person with typical hearing. A person who is functionally deaf does not. So, grouping children who are deaf and children who are hard of hearing into a single educational program does both an unfortunate disservice (i.e., the hard of hearing child is often put into an intervention program that has a visual emphasis, due to the inaccurate assumption that the child who is hard of hearing is most like the child who is deaf).

In this new millennium, the degree of hearing loss ought not determine the functional outcome for infants and children who are young enough to have brain neural plasticity; these children's auditory brain centers can be accessed, stimulated, and developed through the early use of amplification or cochlear implant technologies. A primary desired outcome of auditory-verbal intervention is to enable children who are audiometrically deaf to be functionally hard of hearing (hearing) rather than functionally deaf (visual). The reality is that being functionally hard of hearing accesses the auditory centers of the brain, and that critical auditory brain access opens a world of choices and opportunity for listening and learning.

Note that most traditional and current early intervention programs for children with hearing impairments, even oral programs, have a visual emphasis ("watch me") based on the assumption that the mere presence of a hearing loss prevents a child from learning auditorally ("listen to me"). As you will read in Chapter One, with appropriate technology and auditory-verbal communication at a young age, a child with even profound audiometric deafness can learn spoken language and reading skills on a par with their hearing peers, through accessing the auditory centers of the brain (Robertson & Flexer, 1993).

Hearing Loss

TYPES OF HEARING IMPAIRMENT
Hearing impairments are caused by damage or disease in the auditory system. Based on the location of the damage, called the "site of lesion," there are three general types of hearing impairments: conductive, sensorineural, and mixed (Stach, 1998). A conductive hearing loss occurs when the damage is located in the outer and/or the middle ear. The most common conductive-type hearing losses in young children are caused by *otitis media* (ear infections) (Pappas, 1998). Conductive hearing losses often can be "fixed" by medical or surgical intervention. A sensorineural hearing loss occurs in the tiny, intricate inner ear called the cochlea. Most often, the delicate hair cells (sensory receptor cells) are affected, and sometimes the auditory cranial nerve also is affected. The inner ear might not have developed fully in the first place, or it may have been damaged by disease, lack of oxygen, noise, or medications. Sensorineural hearing losses cannot be fixed by medicines or surgery.

TIME OF ONSET OF HEARING IMPAIRMENT
Hearing impairments in children can be classified into congenital and acquired hearing losses relative to when in the child's life the hearing impairment first occurs (Northern & Downs, 1991). *Congenital hearing impairments* typically occur before, at, or shortly after birth but prior to the learning of speech and language — usually before the age of 3. In contrast, *acquired hearing impairments* occur after speech and language have developed. The negative effects of an acquired hearing impairment tend to be less severe than those of a congenital hearing impairment because the brain already has been programmed for auditory language, spoken communication, and reading.

GENERAL CAUSES OF HEARING IMPAIRMENT
Both congenital and acquired hearing impairments can be caused by *endogenous* or *exogenous* factors (Pappas, 1998). Endogenous hearing impairments are genetic (hereditary) and they have different probabilities of occurrence. On the other hand, exogenous hearing impairments are caused by external and not genetic events. Therefore, exogenous hearing impairments cannot be transmitted to offspring; they include agents such as bacterial or viral infections, noise exposure and medications that can damage the inner ear. At least 50% of congenital hearing impairments have no identifiable cause, and it's speculated that about 90% of hearing impairments with no known cause are genetic in origin (Pappas, 1998).

SEVERITY OR DEGREE OF HEARING IMPAIRMENT: AN AUDIOMETRIC PERSPECTIVE

In addition to being classified by cause and time of onset, hearing impairments also can be categorized by severity, by how much the hearing impairment blocks an infant's sound reception. Degree of hearing loss is determined by looking at an audiogram.

Children with *normal hearing sensitivity* are able to distinguish sound intensities of 15 dB HL (decibels in Hearing Level) or softer in a quiet room. Details of all speech sounds are available, provided that the environment is acoustically accessible. Note that the cut-off for normal hearing sensitivity for children is 15 dB HL.

A *minimal or slight hearing impairment* for children occurs from 16 dB HL to 25 dB HL. A child with an unmanaged minimal hearing impairment may experience problems hearing faint or distant speech, detecting subtle conversational cues, keeping up with fast-paced communicative interactions and hearing the word–sound distinctions (such as *s, ed, ing*) that comprise the meaning for tense, plurality, possessives, and so on. Psychosocial adjustment and academic progression can be negatively influenced by a minimal hearing loss (Bess, Dodd-Murphy, & Parker, 1998). Thus, some form of amplification technology (hearing aids or FM systems) is needed by children who experience minimal hearing losses.

A *mild hearing impairment* occurs from 26 dB HL to 40 dB HL. Without audiologic management, a child who experiences a 30 dB hearing impairment can miss 25%–40% of the speech signal depending on the noise level in the room and the distance from the speaker. Without the use of hearing technology, the child who has a 35 dB–40 dB hearing impairment can miss up to 50% of class discussions.

A *moderate hearing impairment* occurs from 41 dB HL to 55 dB HL. Prior to effective hearing management, a child with a moderate hearing impairment might understand face-to-face conversational speech at a distance of 3–5 feet if content, topic, and vocabulary are known; 50%–75% of the speech signal can be missed with a 40 dB–45 dB hearing impairment, and 80%–100% might be missed with a 50 dB hearing impairment. Without amplification and intervention, the child is likely to have a limited vocabulary and imperfect speech production.

A *moderately-severe hearing impairment* occurs from 56 dB HL to 70 dB HL. If amplification technologies are not used, spoken communication must be very loud and very close to be minimally understood.

A *severe hearing impairment* occurs from 71 dB HL to 90 dB HL and will prevent a child from hearing all conversational speech without amplification. With early and appropriate amplification, that child should be able to detect all speech sounds as well as environmental sounds — but not at great distances. And, the child needs to have therapy/intervention to learn the meaning of incoming sounds.

A *profound hearing impairment* means that the hearing loss is 91 dB HL or worse. A person with a profound hearing loss cannot hear any sounds without amplification. However, very few people have absolutely no residual hearing. The vast majority of persons with profound hearing impairments do have some residual or remaining hearing. An infant or child with a profound hearing loss should be referred for a cochlear implant evaluation; a cochlear implant could provide much better sound access to the brain than hearing aids (Estabrooks, 1998).

People with hearing losses in the minimal to moderately severe range can be described as being *audiometrically hard of hearing*. That is, they have some brain access and stimulation from sound in the environment even without using amplification technology — although we would never leave a person without technology. Persons with hearing losses in the severe to profound range are described as being *audiometrically deaf*. A person who is audiometrically deaf has no access to sounds in the environment — they receive no auditory neural stimulation — until they use amplification technology or cochlear implants. Before we had high quality amplification, cochlear implants and early auditory intervention, the degree of hearing loss was indeed the primary determiner of functional outcome. The greater the degree of hearing loss, the more visual the person typically needed to be. However, in this new millennium, degree of hearing loss ought not determine functional outcome, provided we identify the hearing loss early, and, through hearing aids and cochlear implants, direct acoustic detail to critical auditory brain centers.

The more functionally hard of hearing a child who is audiometrically hard of hearing or deaf becomes, the better their opportunity for literacy development. Note the distinction between *audiometric definitions* of hard of hearing and deaf (degree of hearing loss as noted on an audiogram), and *functional definitions* of hard of hearing (primarily auditory in orientation with subsequent auditory brain development) and deaf (primarily visual in orientation with limited auditory brain development).

Mark Ross and colleagues make one final point. He writes that the quality and integrity of the audiologic management that a baby/child receives from the beginning, is the greatest single factor in determining if a child will be functionally hard of hearing, or functionally deaf (Ross, Brackett, & Maxon, 1991). *Families need to find an aggressive pediatric audiologist who can access and stimulate critical auditory brain centers through early and appropriate fitting of amplification technologies.*

ACOUSTIC FILTER EFFECT OF HEARING IMPAIRMENT

Hearing loss of any type or degree that occurs in infancy or childhood can interfere with the development of a child's spoken language, reading and writing skills, and academic performance (Davis, 1990; Ling, 1989). That is, hearing loss can be described as an *invisible acoustic filter* that distorts, smears, or eliminates incoming sounds, especially sounds from a distance — even a short distance. The negative effects of a hearing loss may be apparent, but the hearing loss itself is invisible and easily ignored or underestimated.

It is critical to note that as human beings we are neurologically "wired" to develop spoken language (speech) and reading skills through the central *auditory* system. Most people think that reading is a visual skill, but recent research on brain mapping shows that primary reading centers of the brain are located in the auditory cortex — in the auditory portions of the brain (Chermak & Musiek, 1997). That is why many children who are born with hearing losses and who do not have access to auditory input when they are very young (through strong hearing aids and auditory teaching), tend to have a great deal of difficulty reading even though their vision is fine. Therefore, the earlier and more efficiently we can allow a child access to meaningful sound with subsequent direction of the child's attention to sound, the better opportunity that child will have to develop spoken language, literacy, and academic skills. *With the technology and early auditory intervention available today, a child with a hearing loss CAN have the same opportunity as a typically hearing child to develop spoken language, reading and academic skills.*

AUDIBILITY/INTELLIGIBILITY DISTINCTIONS

There is a big difference between an "audible" signal and an "intelligible" signal. Speech is audible if the person is able simply to detect its presence. However, for speech to be intelligible, the person must be able to discriminate the word–sound distinctions of individual phonemes or speech sounds. As Mark Ross has said often, the major problem with having a hearing loss is that you cannot hear so good! Consequently, speech might be very audible but not consistently intelligible to a child with even a minimal hearing loss, causing the child to hear, for example, words such as "walked," "walking," "walker," and "walks," all as "___ah."

Vowel sounds (such as *o, u, ee,* etc.) are low frequency sounds and they are the most powerful sounds in English; they cause speech to be audible. Consonant sounds (like *sh* and *s*) are high frequency sounds and are much weaker; consonants allow speech to be intelligible. For speech to be heard clearly, both vowels and consonants must be acoustically available. Persons with hearing losses typically have the most difficulty hearing the weak, high frequency consonant sounds.

"Computer Analogy" and Amplification Technology

One way to illustrate the potentially negative effects of any type and degree of hearing impairment on a child's language and overall development and to explain the role of amplification technology, is to use a computer analogy. The primary concept is: *data input precedes data processing.*

An infant or toddler (or anyone) must have information/data in order to learn. A primary avenue for entering information into the brain is through the ears, via hearing. So, the ears can be thought of as analogous to a computer keyboard, and the brain could be compared to a computer "hard drive." Remember, as human beings we are neurologically wired to code and, hence, to develop spoken language and reading skills through the auditory centers of the brain; the hard drive (Northern & Downs, 1991). Therefore, auditory data input is critical, and it is worth our time and effort to make detailed auditory information available to a child with any degree of hearing loss. If data are entered inaccurately, incompletely, or inconsistently, analogous to using a malfunctioning computer keyboard or to having one's fingers on the wrong keys of a computer keyboard, the child's brain or hard drive will have incorrect or incomplete information to process. How can a child be expected to learn when the information that reaches his or her brain is deficient? Amplification technology such as hearing aids, personal FM systems or sound-field FM systems, and biomedical devices such as cochlear implants can all be thought of as keyboards — as a means of entering acoustic information into the child's hard drive. So, all that technology is, really, is a more efficient keyboard. Unfortunately, technology is not a perfect keyboard and it does not have a life of its own, anymore than a car has a life of its own. Technology is only as effective as the use to which it is put, and only as efficient as the people who use it. Conversely, without the technology, without acoustic data input, auditory brain access is not possible for persons with hearing impairment.

To continue the computer analogy, once the keyboard is repaired or the figurative "fingers" are placed on the correct keys of the keyboard — allowing data to be entered accurately, analogous to using amplification technology that enables a child to detect word–sound distinctions — what happens to all of the previously entered inaccurate and incomplete information? Is there a magic button that automatically converts inaccurate data to complete and correct information? Unfortunately, all of the corrected data need to be re-entered. Thus, the longer a child's hearing problem remains unrecognized and unmanaged, the more destructive and far-reaching are the snowballing effects of hearing impairment. *Early intervention is critical — the earlier the better!*

Hearing is only the *first* step in the intervention chain. Once hearing has been accessed as much as possible through appropriate amplification or biomedical technology, the child will have an opportunity to discriminate word–sound distinctions as a basis for learning language, which in turn provides the child with an opportunity to communicate and acquire knowledge of the world. All levels of the acoustic filter effect of hearing impairment discussed previously need to be understood and managed. In other words, just wearing hearing aids or a cochlear implant does not ensure development of an effective language base.

The longer a child's data entry is inaccurate, the more damaging the snowballing acoustic filter effects will be on the child's overall life development. Conversely the more intelligible and complete the data entered are, the better opportunity the infant or toddler will have to learn language that serves as a foundation for later reading and academic skills. *It can't be said enough — early intervention is critical!*

The point is, from the inception of early intervention programming, comprehensive audiologic and hearing management is an absolutely necessary first step for a child of any age with any type of hearing or listening difficulty to have an opportunity to learn.

A critical caveat is that, although amplification technology can provide a better "keyboard", a more efficient and consistent route of data entry, that keyboard will not be perfect. Thus, listening and learning strategies also need to be implemented; hence the importance of auditory-verbal intervention.

The exciting news is that a cochlear implant can provide a much more complete and efficient keyboard than can hearing aids for a child who is audiometrically deaf, even if that child is obtaining some benefit from hearing aids and FM systems.

Distance Hearing

Children with hearing losses, even minimal ones, cannot receive intelligible speech well over distances. This reduction in "earshot" has tremendous negative consequences for life and classroom performance because distance hearing is linked to passive/casual/incidental listening and learning. Research in the field of developmental psychology tells us that about 90% of what very young children know about spoken language and the world, they learn incidentally (Flexer, 1999). That is, young children learn a great deal of information unintentionally because they have access to overhearing conversations that occur at distances. Thus, any type and degree of hearing loss can present a significant barrier to an infant or child's ability to receive information from the environment.

Because of the reduction in acoustic signal intensity and integrity with distance, a child with a hearing problem has a limited range or distance hearing; that child may need to be taught directly many skills that other children learn incidentally.

Understanding Audiograms

An audiologist is the specialist who obtains an audiogram. An audiologist is a professional who holds a graduate degree (Master's or doctorate) in audiology and specializes in the assessment and management of hearing and hearing problems. Audiology is to hearing as optometry is to vision. Most states require a license to practice audiology. Because some audiologists specialize in pediatric evaluation and management, it is important to ask whether yours has had experience with children. Note that physicians specialize in medical and surgical management of disease; an audiologist specializes in the diagnosis and management (i.e., fitting hearing aids, FM devices, mapping cochlear implants) of hearing problems.

It is important to know that an infant of any age can be evaluated by a qualified pediatric audiologist. There is NO need to wait for an audiometric evaluation if you suspect any hearing difficulties. Parents should be included in all audiometric test sessions to participate in the diagnosis because they are key members of the team.

An audiogram is a simple graph that charts what a person can hear (see Figure 1). The audiogram is produced by testing a person in a sound-isolated booth using pure tones presented through headphones or through insert earphones (Stach, 1998). This hearing test — the professional term is audiologic evaluation performed by an audiologist — demonstrates how loud a sound needs to be for a person to just barely hear it.

An audiogram shows the type of hearing loss (conductive, sensorineural, or mixed), the degree of hearing loss (ranging from minimal to profound), and the pattern of the hearing loss (how much hearing loss exists at different frequencies).

Frequencies from 250 Hz through 8000 Hz are shown along the horizontal dimension. The low-pitched sounds are 250 Hz and 500 Hz; they have a bass quality and carry the melody of speech, vowel sounds, and most environmental sounds. It is important to note that 90% of the energy of speech (audibility) is carried in the lower frequencies. High-pitched sounds, on the other hand, have frequencies above 1500 Hz and have a tenor quality. High-frequency sounds are very important for hearing speech because they carry the energy involved in consonant production (such as s, sh, f, and th). That is, high frequencies carry the meaning of speech (intelligibility), whereas low frequencies, primarily, carry the melody. Only 10% of the energy of speech but 90% of the meaning is carried by the higher frequencies.

Intensity or loudness in dB HL is displayed along the vertical dimension of the audiogram. The higher the number of decibels, the louder the sound. There is approximately a 30 dB range between the softest and most powerful speech sounds throughout the frequency range. The weakest, least intense speech sound is the voiceless *th* as in "thin." The strongest, most intense speech sound is *ah* as in "law."

Threshold is defined as the softest sound that the person can hear. All sounds greater or louder than threshold (toward the bottom of the graph) are audible. Sounds softer than threshold (toward the top of the graph) are not audible.

The threshold of sensitivity for each ear is displayed on an audiogram using the following symbols:

1. O = the softest sound that the person can hear with his or her right ear under headphones.
2. X = the softest sound that the person can hear with his or her left ear under headphones.
3. ^ = the softest sound that the person can hear when being tested by bone conduction; the test ear is not specified.
4. S = sound-field thresholds. The tones are presented through loudspeakers directly into the sound room. Sound-field thresholds often are obtained when a baby or young child will not wear headphones or when a comparison is needed between hearing aided and unaided tones.
5. A = aided sound-field thresholds — the softest sounds that a person can hear while wearing hearing aids. Whenever a child wears hearing aids, sound-field aided measurements must be made to determine how the child is functioning with amplification in the real world. A child's aided sensitivity cannot be known without obtaining data. It is therefore important to include aided as well as unaided thresholds on a child's audiogram to compare, according to acoustic phonetics, speech sounds that are audible with and without amplification.
6. C = cochlear implant thresholds — the softest sounds that a person can hear while wearing their cochlear implant. The same considerations discussed under "aided thresholds" apply here, also.

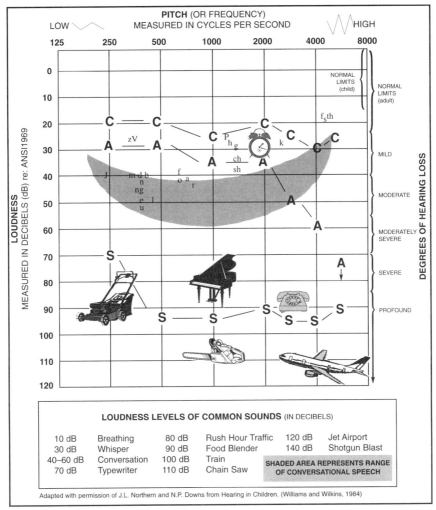

Adapted with permission of J.L. Northern and N.P. Downs from Hearing in Children. (Williams and Wilkins, 1984)

Figure I.1. This audiogram (graph of an individual's hearing sensitivity) shows not only frequency (pitch) and intensity (loudness) but also the relationship of both to specific speech and environmental sounds. On this audiogram, aided thresholds (A) show the softest tones that the child could hear when she wore hearing aids, as compared with cochlear implant thresholds (C) which show the softest sounds that she now can hear with her new cochlear implant. Both aided and cochlear implant thresholds are compared with unaided sound-field thresholds (S) that show the softest sounds the child can hear without technology of any kind. This child has profound audiometric deafness, but she functions as a child who is hard of hearing due to early identification, aggressive use of hearing aids, and then cochlear implant technology and auditory-verbal intervention. Even though she obtained benefit from her hearing aids, she has qualitatively and quantitatively better auditory brain access with her cochlear implant.

In the new millennium, when properly fitted with amplification technologies or a cochlear implant, a child with any degree of hearing loss ought to be able to detect the entire speech spectrum at a soft conversational level of loudness.

Amplification Technologies

Amplification technologies are the key to successful use of auditory input for persons with all types and degrees of hearing loss, including sensorineural hearing loss. Some people are told that amplification technology will not help children with sensorineural hearing losses; that statement is false. Technology enables persons with hearing losses to hear sounds that they could not hear at all without amplification; technology gets sound to the auditory centers of the brain. As technology with subsequent brain access improves, children's opportunities for auditory learning and literacy also improve.

HEARING OR LISTENING AGE

A critical concept that pertains to the attainment of spoken language and literacy skills is the notion of hearing or listening age. A child's auditory-language development begins when amplification technology is first used (Estabrooks, 1998). If a child is 2 years old when her hearing loss is identified, she is one day old relative to listening, language, and information learning when her hearing aids are first fit or when her cochlear implant is activated and mapped. So, when that child reaches age 3, chronologically, she is 1 year old relative to her hearing and learning experiences; she will sound and behave linguistically and socially more like a 1-year old than a 3-year old. Her *listening* age is 1 year. There is nothing wrong with a child who shows this discrepancy; she hasn't had much time for "data to be entered." This expected gap between a child's chronological and listening age decreases over time, *provided* that the child uses appropriate amplification technology during all waking hours, and has active family-centered auditory intervention. In addition, the earlier a child's hearing problem is identified and managed, the smaller the gap will be from the outset. Time is not on our side relative to brain neural plasticity!

SENSORY DEPRIVATION

The longer the brain is deprived of auditory input, the greater the resultant sensory deprivation. *Sensory deprivation* is lack of sensory stimulation to the brain due to a hearing impairment (Northern & Downs, 1991). Not only does sensory deprivation prevent the occurrence of auditory learning, deprivation also prevents neural growth and development. The longer the deprivation, the more "stunted" is auditory brain growth. In fact, not only will auditory centers not grow, but existing "pre-wired" auditory tracts can degenerate. So, if we wait too long to access the brain through technology, auditory brain centers may not be available to respond to input. Early intervention is critical! (Yoshinaga-Itano, Sedey, Coulter, & Mehl, 1998).

THE LISTENING ENVIRONMENT

The purpose of wearing amplification technology and implementing the auditory-verbal approach is to learn spoken language through listening rather than watching. Conversations, therapy, and education must therefore be carried out in the best possible listening conditions to make information easy to hear. The acoustic environment can be enhanced by: minimizing background noise (turn off the TV and stereo); speaking close to the child at a regular vocal volume; and using speech that is rich in melody, expression and rhythm and that is repetitive.

SPEECH-TO-NOISE RATIO (ALSO CALLED SIGNAL-TO-NOISE RATIO)

The Signal-to-Noise (S/N) ratio is the relationship between the primary speech or input signal and background noise (Berg, 1993). Background noise is anything and everything that interferes with the reception of the desired auditory signal and includes other talkers, heating or cooling systems, home and classroom sounds, television, computers, wind, traffic noise, internal biological sounds, etc. The more favorable the S/N ratio (the louder the desired auditory signal relative to background sounds), the more intelligible the speech or auditory signal will be for the child. An intelligible speech signal provides children with a better opportunity to learn the word–sound differences that underlie the development of spoken communication.

People with normal hearing typically require an S/N ratio of +6 dB for the reception of intelligible speech; speech needs to be about twice as loud as competing sounds. Due to the auditory distortion of the hearing loss itself, persons with a hearing problem need an S/N ratio of +20 dB; speech needs to be about 10 times louder than background sounds. Due to reverberation, noise, and changes in teacher position, the average classroom S/N ratio is only about +4 dB, and it may be 0 dB, which is less than ideal even for children with normal hearing (Berg, 1993).

One strategy for improving the S/N ratio is to move closer to the infant or child's ear so that the speaker's voice will take precedence over all background sounds. Yelling from across the room promotes only audibility, not intelligibility, whereas an average loudness of speech very close to the ear facilitates intelligibility of the speech signal. Sitting across from a child does not produce as favorable a S/N as sitting next to a child.

HEARING AIDS

Hearing aids — miniature public address systems — typically are the initial technology used to enhance the reception of sound for an individual who has a hearing impairment. Hearing aids do not correct the hearing impairment; rather, they function to amplify and shape the incoming sounds to make them audible to the child. Once sounds are detected by a child, he or she must then have rich, meaningful listening experiences to learn to make sense of the new incoming sounds. Hearing aids can be fitted on infants as young as 1–3 months old. Appropriate fitting of hearing aids on children is a complex and ongoing process (Flexer, 1999). It is important to work with a pediatric audiologist. Please see suggested readings at the end of this Introduction for additional information about hearing aids.

FM UNITS OR FM AUDITORY TRAINERS

Hearing aids are not designed to deal with all listening needs (Flexer, 1997). Their biggest limitation is their inability to enhance the S/N ratio in situations where the listener cannot be physically close to the speaker. Because a clear and complete speech signal is essential for the development of oral expressive language, some means must be provided to enhance the S/N ratio. An FM unit is such a device.

An FM unit is a personal listening device that includes a remote microphone placed near the desired sound source, and a receiver for the listener who can be situated anywhere within 50 to 500 feet. No wires are required to connect the speaker and listener because the unit is really a small FM radio that transmits and receives on a single frequency. Because the talker wears the remote microphone within six inches of his of her mouth, the personal FM unit creates a listening situation that is comparable to the parent, teacher, or therapist being six inches from the child's ear at all times, thereby allowing for a positive and constant S/N ratio.

An FM unit can be attached to a child's hearing aid, or worn instead of a hearing aid. Once again, it is important to work with a pediatric audiologist to find the most appropriate FM unit for the child. *We recommend that FM units be fitted on babies and children at the same time as hearing aids, and that they be used at home as well as in school to enhance speech intelligibility, distance hearing and incidental learning* (Flexer, 1997).

SOUND-FIELD FM SYSTEMS

Personal FM units are worn by the individual and the talker and can be used anywhere. Sound-field FM units are classroom devices. Basically, sound-field FM units provide amplification for the entire classroom through the use of two, three, or four wall or ceiling-mounted loudspeakers (Crandell, Smaldino & Flexer, 1995). All students in the room benefit from an improved S/N ratio of approximately +10 dB to +20 dB no matter where they or the teacher are positioned. Sound-field FM systems show exciting promise for providing children, whether or not they have hearing problems, with better access to intelligible speech and hence, enhances their reading and learning.

COCHLEAR IMPLANTS

A cochlear implant is a biomedical device that is designed to provide sound information to children and adults who are profoundly hearing impaired (Tucker, 1998). The cochlear implant is not like a hearing aid. In fact, the implant bypasses the damaged hair cells of the inner ear. Coded electrical signals are sent through a tiny electrode array that is surgically inserted in the cochlea by a neuro-otologist. The signals stimulate different hearing nerve fibers, which then send auditory information to the brain. A cochlear implant, therefore, is a "treatment" for severe to profound sensorineural hearing impairment.

The cochlear implant opens a new frontier of sound for children with audiometric deafness. A cochlear implant, if implemented when the child is very young and if auditory-verbal communication and intervention is emphasized, can in our opinion, enable a child to function like a child with a moderate hearing loss who is well amplified; like a child who is hard of hearing.

OUR OBSERVATIONS REGARDING COCHLEAR IMPLANT CANDIDACY ISSUES AS THEY RELATE TO CHILDREN WHO HAVE RECEIVED AUDITORY-VERBAL INTERVENTION

My audiological criteria for cochlear implant eligibility include a desired outcome for that child of spoken language, reading and academic skills consistent with hearing peers; mainstream placement; unaided thresholds of 90 dB or worse from 750 Hz through 8000 Hz; aided distance hearing less than 10 feet for /s/, and less than 20 feet for /sh/; some difficulty following an open-set communicative exchange with two people; and an aided SRT of 35 dB HL or worse. If children who have been receiving auditory-verbal communication intervention meet these criteria, I refer them for a cochlear implant evaluation, even though they are benefiting from their hearing aids and are using their hearing in a functional and productive way. It should be noted that an older child with a profound hearing loss who has never had auditory brain stimulation would be a questionable implant candidate due to sensory deprivation.

Why would I refer children with profound hearing losses for cochlear implants even if they are receiving benefit from amplification? Because they could receive greater and easier acoustic access with a cochlear implant. Why should auditory-verbal children be denied a better technology (cochlear implants) just because they have had extensive therapy and have learned to use the more limited auditory cues provided by their hearing aids? That is, the cochlea of an auditory-verbally taught child with a profound hearing loss is not more intact than the cochlea of a visually taught child with a profound hearing loss. The auditory advantage for the auditory-verbal child is in the high expectation of the ability to use hearing, extensive use of technology, and auditory-based rather than visually-based teaching. In fact, the more auditory focus and the more auditory experience a child has had with their hearing aids prior to receiving a cochlear implant, the faster and more efficiently they can progress after they receive their implant. Why? Because their brain has already been "programmed" with auditory information. Using the computer analogy, their "hard drive" is available to receive the more complete auditory information provided through the "keyboard" of a cochlear implant.

Auditory-Verbal Communication and Intervention for Children with Hearing Impairments

Early identification of hearing loss with subsequent effective fitting of amplification technology is the first step in intervention. Once acoustic detail is directed to auditory brain centers, the child then must be taught to listen and distinguish the auditory events of spoken language and environmental sounds.

Auditory-verbal is a model of communication and intervention for children with hearing impairments that incorporates the principles adapted from Doreen Pollack and listed in Chapter One. These guiding principles outline the essential requirements needed to enable young children with hearing impairments to use even minimal amounts of amplified residual hearing to learn to listen, to process spoken language, and to speak. The desired outcome of auditory-verbal intervention is that children with all degrees of hearing loss can grow up in typical learning and living environments using amplified hearing and spoken language that enables them to become independent and contributing adults.

Note that auditory-verbal is not merely a "technique" to be delivered 2 hours a week, but rather a way of life to be practiced on a daily basis. Consequently, professionals require specialized training and certification to deliver auditory-verbal services. Even though auditory-verbal therapists have had special training, it is not the teacher contact hours that matter; it is the parent contact. Therapy is not really designed to teach the child at all, but rather to assess the child's progress toward developmentally appropriate auditory (listening), cognitive (thinking), and speech targets. Parents attend every therapy session and participate in practice activities that enable them to constantly integrate targets at home. *The goal is that auditory brain centers will be richly developed, enabling the child who is audiometrically deaf to be functionally hard of hearing with speech, reading, and academic potential equal to hearing peers.*

Concept of "Desired Outcome" — Evaluating the Success of an Intervention or Amplification Technology Relative to the Desired Outcome of that Technology

One important way of defining "success" and of evaluating the efficacy of an amplification and/or treatment strategy is to examine that treatment's social validity; is the desired long-range outcome actually achieved? The desired outcome needs to be specified and then the attainment of that outcome needs to be evaluated. For example, if the desired and targeted outcomes for a child with a hearing impairment include the development of efficient and effective spoken language, age-appropriate reading skills, and integration and independent function in mainstream classrooms and in the community as a person who is functionally "hard of hearing," then that treatment would have been successful if those desired outcomes have been achieved. Research studies by Goldberg and Flexer (1993), and Robertson and Flexer (1993) document that these specified desired outcomes for auditory-verbal intervention are possible.

The "success" of a technology such as hearing aids, FM systems, cochlear implants, or of a model of intervention such as auditory-verbal, is not a matter of good or bad or of right or wrong. Success can be defined logically in terms of attaining specified desired outcomes. Who defines desired outcomes? For young children, the parents set the vision for the desired outcome.

Listening Skill Development

Children, with or without a hearing loss, are not able to "listen" like adults. The auditory neural network of a child is not as developed as that of an adult because the higher cortical areas of the brain are not fully mature until a child is about 15 years old. In addition, children do not bring years of language and world experience to a listening situation; thus, children cannot perform auditory/cognitive closure of missed information.

There are data to suggest that listening experience (having access to the language sounds in the world) also may be important for all children in terms of influencing the spatial organization and richness of their auditory cortex, especially in the early years of brain neural plasticity (Boothroyd, 1997; Musiek & Berge, 1998). If spatial organization of the auditory cortex is influenced by the properties of the acoustic environment in which an infant is raised, then enriching the auditory environment causes enrichment of the auditory brain centers (Sharpe, 1994). Therefore, meaningful sounds must be routinely and efficiently channeled into the auditory system through management of acoustic/learning environments, the judicious use of hearing aids, cochlear implants and S/N ratio-enhancing technology. [See Table 1 for some suggestions for providing listening and auditory language enrichment for your child as a way of life.]

A child who has a hearing loss should be able to "hear" (receive sounds) better with hearing aids than without them. Unfortunately, amplification alone does not necessarily ensure that the child will be better able to "listen," just as having normal hearing does not guarantee the development of listening skills.

Unless a purposeful attempt is made to teach the child what to listen for, the only goal that may be achieved with amplification is to increase the volume of sounds that are heard. A child must be provided with opportunities to learn the meaning of incoming sounds. The focus is not on pointless, isolated auditory training sessions that occur twice weekly for 20 minutes, but rather on integrating listening skills and spoken communication into daily life (i.e., auditory living, not mere auditory training). Listening skills are not separate from learning, but are the means of learning.

Conclusion

The purpose of this Introduction has been to provide an overview of hearing loss, amplification technologies, cochlear implants, auditory-verbal communication and listening skill development. Hearing is a first-order event for the development of spoken language and literacy skills. *The building and enrichment of critical auditory brain centers creates the neurological foundation for literacy.*

Please refer to the list of suggested readings at the end of this Introduction for more in-depth information about audiology, amplification technology, cochlear implants, listening skill development and auditory-verbal communication.

Table I.1. How to Provide Active Listening and Auditory-Based Language Enrichment for Your Child Every Day

1. The *quieter* the room and the *closer* you are to your child, the better you will be heard. Remember, your child may have difficulty "overhearing" conversations and hearing you from a distance. You need to be close to your child when you speak.

2. Your child must *wear his or her hearing aid or cochlear implant during all waking hours* (except bathing or swimming, of course), every day of the week. The brain needs constant, detailed auditory input in order to develop.

3. *Use an FM system at home* to facilitate distance hearing and incidental learning. An FM system can be used during reading, too, to improve the signal-to-noise ratio and to facilitate the development of auditory self monitoring.

4. *Focus on listening,* not just seeing. Call attention to sounds and to conversations in the room.

5. *Maintain a joint focus of attention* when reading and when engaged in activities. That is, the child looks at the book or at the activity while listening to you.

6. Speak in sentences, not single words, with *clear speech* using lots of melody.

7. *Read aloud* to your child, daily. Even infants can be read to, as can older children. Try to read at least 10 books to your baby or child each day.

8. *Sing and read nursery rhymes* to your baby or young child every day.

9. Name *objects* in the environment as you encounter them during daily routines. Constantly be mindful of expanding vocabulary.

10. Talk about and *describe* how things sound, look, and feel.

11. Talk about where objects are *located.* You will use many prepositions such as in, on, under, behind, beside, next to, between.

12. Compare how objects or actions are *similar and different* in size, shape, quantity, smell, color, and texture.

13. *Describe sequences.* Talk about the steps involved in activities as you are doing the activity.

14. Tell *familiar stories* or stories about events from your day or from your past. Keep *narratives* simpler for younger children, and increase complexity as your child grows.

Suggested Reading

Amplification Technology (Hearing Aids and FM Systems)

Bess, F.G., Gravel, J.S., & Tharpe, A.M. (Eds.) (1996). *Amplification for children with auditory deficits.* Nashville, TN: Bill Wilkerson Center Press.

Flexer, C. (1997). Individual and sound-field FM systems: Rationale, description, and use. *The Volta Review,* 99(3), 133-162.

Flexer, C. (1998). Enhancing classrooms for listening, language and literacy. [Videotape] (Available from Alexander Graham Bell Association for the Deaf and Hard of Hearing, Washington, DC.)

Tye Murray, N. (1998). *Foundations of aural rehabilitation.* San Diego, CA: Singular Publishing Group.

Audiology

Flexer, C. (1999). *Facilitating hearing and listening in young children* (2nd. ed.). San Diego, CA: Singular Publishing Group.

Martin, F.N., & Clark, J.G. (1996). *Hearing care for children.* Boston: Allyn and Bacon.

Stach, B.A. (1998). *Clinical audiology: An introduction.* San Diego, CA: Singular Publishing Group.

Auditory-Verbal Practice and Listening Skill Development

Estabrooks, W. (Ed.) (1994). *Auditory-verbal therapy for parents and professionals.* Washington, DC: Alexander Graham Bell Association for the Deaf and Hard of Hearing.

Parents and Families of Natural Communication, Inc. (1998). *We CAN hear and speak! The power of auditory-verbal communication for children who are deaf or hard of hearing.* Washington, DC: Alexander Graham Bell Association for the Deaf and Hard of Hearing.

Pollack, D., Goldberg, D., & Caleffe-Schenck, N. (1997). *Educational audiology for the limited-hearing infant and preschooler: An auditory verbal program* (3rd ed.). Springfield, IL: Charles C. Thomas.

Sindrey, D. (1997). *Listening games for littles.* London, Ontario, Canada: Word Play Publications.

Cochlear Implants

Estabrooks, W. (Ed.) (1998). *Cochlear implants for kids.* Washington, DC: Alexander Graham Bell Association for the Deaf and Hard of Hearing.

Tucker, B. (1998). *Cochlear implants: A handbook.* Jefferson, NC: McFarland & Company, Inc.

References

Berg, F.S. (1993). *Acoustics and sound systems in schools.* San Diego, CA: Singular Publishing Group.

Bess, F.H., Dodd-Murphy, J., & Parker, R.A. (1998). Children with minimal sensorineural hearing loss: prevalence, educational performance, and functional status. *Ear and Hearing,* 19, 339-354.

Boothroyd, A. (1997). Auditory development of the hearing child. *Scandinavian Audiology,* 26(Suppl. 46), 9-16.

Boutte, V. (1998). A new age for advocacy. *Volta Voices,* 5, 19-21.

Chermak, G.D., & Musiek, F.E. (1997). *Central auditory processing disorders: New perspectives.* San Diego, CA: Singular Publishing Group.

Crandell, C.C., Smaldino, J.J., & Flexer, C. (1995). *Sound-field FM amplification: Theory and practical applications.* San Diego, CA: Singular Publishing Group.

Davis, J. (Ed.) (1990). *Our forgotten children: Hard-of-hearing pupils in the schools.* Bethesda, MD: Self Help for Hard of Hearing People.

Estabrooks, W. (Ed.) (1998). *Cochlear implants for kids.* Washington, DC: Alexander Graham Bell Association for the Deaf and Hard of Hearing.

Flexer, C. (1997). Individual and sound-field FM systems: Rationale, description, and use. *The Volta Review,* 99(3), 133-162.

Flexer, C. (1999). *Facilitating hearing and listening in young children* (2nd ed.). San Diego, CA: Singular Publishing Group.

Gilbertson, M., & Bramlett, R.K. (1998). Phonological awareness screening to identify at-risk readers: Implications for practitioners. *Language, Speech and Hearing Services in Schools,* 29, 109-116.

Goldberg, D.M., & Flexer, C. (1993). Outcome survey of auditory-verbal graduates: Study of clinical efficacy. *Journal of the American Academy of Audiology,* 4, 189-200.

Ling, D. (1989). *Foundations of spoken language for hearing impaired children.* Washington, DC: Alexander Graham Bell Association for the Deaf and Hard of Hearing.

Manning, A. (1998, June 29). Women outpacing men by degrees. *USA Today* (page 1)

Musiek, F.E., & Berge, B.E. (1998). A neuroscience view of auditory training/stimulation and central auditory processing disorders. In M.G. Masters, N.A. Stecker, & J. Katz (Eds.), *Central auditory processing disorders: Mostly management* (pp. 15-32). Boston: Allyn and Bacon.

Northern, J.L., & Downs, M.P. (1991). *Hearing in children* (4th ed.). Baltimore: Williams & Wilkins.

Pappas, D.G. (1998). *Diagnosis and treatment of hearing impairment in children* (2nd ed.). San Diego, CA: Singular Publishing Group.

Robertson, L., & Flexer, C. (1993). Reading development: A parent survey of children with hearing impairment who developed speech and language through the auditory-verbal method. *The Volta Review, 95*(3), 253-261.

Ross, M., Brackett, D., & Maxon, A. (1991). *Assessment and management of mainstreamed hearing-impaired children.* Austin, TX: Pro-Ed.

Sharpe, R., (1994, April 12). The early brain. *Wall Street Journal.*

Stach, B.A. (1998). *Clinical audiology: An introduction.* San Diego, CA: Singular Publishing Group.

Tucker, B.P. (1998). *Cochlear implants: A handbook.* Jefferson, NC: McFarland & Company, Inc.

Yoshinaga-Itano, C. (1998). Early identification and intervention: It does make a difference. *Audiology Today, 10*(Suppl. 11).

Yoshinaga-Itano, C., Sedey A.L., Coulter, D.K., & Mehl, A.L. (1998). Language of early- and later-identified children with hearing loss. *Pediatrics, 102,* 1161-1171.

How Is Hearing Related to Literacy?

Highlights

▼ Deafness and being hard of hearing do not have to be disabilities.

▼ People who are deaf or hard of hearing can develop proficient literacy abilities.

▼ Children who are deaf or hard of hearing who learn their family's spoken language have a good chance of learning to read and to write in that language.

▼ Children who are deaf or hard of hearing can live regular lives alongside schoolmates with normal hearing.

▼ Many children who are deaf or hard of hearing have grown into successful, well-educated adults.

Reading is a Crucial Ability for Getting Along in the World

MY GREATEST WORRY WHEN OUR 15-MONTH-OLD DAUGHTER ANNIE WAS diagnosed with severe-to-profound deafness was that she would never learn how to read and write properly. Because making the connection between spoken and written language is the basis for literacy, I knew it was crucial that she learn the language being spoken, heard, written, and read by the people in her family and her environment. Not knowing the spoken language that is written down makes it impossible to learn to read. Not knowing how to read well enough makes it impossible to thrive, or even just get along, at school. It makes it impossible to take a job with responsibility; it may even make it impossible to take a job at all. The person who cannot read well is simultaneously dependent on and isolated from others in significant ways and is prevented from entering into the simplest of communications with others. Jonathan Kozol (1985) in writing about the population in general points out that literally millions of citizens of the United

States are handicapped severely by the inability to read and write well enough to get along in the simplest of jobs. For the person with a hearing loss, the combination of the inability to read and write with the inability to hear is even more devastating.

The History of Reading Achievement for those with Hearing Loss

The statistics are indeed startling; most people who are deaf or hard of hearing do not acquire reading and writing ability adequate for making their way in the mainstream of society. In using the expression "deaf or hard of hearing," I will be referring throughout this book to loss of hearing anywhere along the continuum from mild to profound loss; however, I am most concerned with children with severe and profound losses because they face the most difficulty in learning spoken language and learning to read and write. When Annie's hearing loss was diagnosed in 1978, I knew about studies as long ago as the one by Pintner and Patterson in 1916 that documented very low reading levels for people who were deaf or hard of hearing. I knew that, in spite of years of attempts to improve literacy levels, more recent studies had demonstrated the same discouraging results. In 1974, Lane and Baker had reported lags of two to five years for children who were deaf or hard of hearing compared to children with normal hearing.

As we proceeded with our own work with Annie, the dismal reports kept coming. Allen (1986) showed 18-year-olds in both 1974 and 1983 at just below third grade level, and Schildroth and Karchmer (1986) found an average of third grade reading level in a group of 15- to 18-year-olds they studied. On a more hopeful note, Geers and Moog (1985) published a report of an experimental educational program that brought 16 10-year-olds to a fourth-grade reading level; and in 1989, they reported on 100 16- and 17-year-olds with profound hearing loss who read at an average eighth-grade level — a full five grade levels above average for individuals who are deaf or hard of hearing. Unfortunately, though, "the majority of the subjects still did not achieve reading levels commensurate with normal-hearing adolescents at the end of high school" (Geers and Moog, 1989).

Seeking a Better Outcome

Working from the premise that learning the spoken language of the family into which she was born would facilitate our daughter's learning to read and to write, we set out to help her accomplish this goal. We tried to inform ourselves about every approach available and settled on the Auditory-Verbal approach after meeting an articulate young high school student with a profound hearing loss who had grown up as a student of Helen Beebe's. In this approach, every effort is made to help the child use her or his residual hearing in order to learn language. I'll describe this approach more fully as these pages unfold.

As parents, we saw our job as helping Annie learn to listen and speak and thereby creating the foundation for her learning to read and write. We lived hundreds of miles from the Helen Beebe Speech and Hearing Center, and so we traveled there, first at six-month intervals and then once a year to soak up everything we could to help us in our task. We also took Annie to weekly sessions with a local speech therapist who was not an auditory-verbal practitioner and enrolled her with the school's speech therapist beginning in kindergarten. Mainly, we talked with Annie and listened to her. We made sure her hearing aids were working as well as technologically possible and sent her to our local public school and to gymnastics, T-ball, and other childhood activities where she would have many children and adults to talk with and listen to.

At the age of 22, Annie reads and writes better than the average person with normal hearing of her age group as judged by standardized tests, including the Scholastic Achievement Test (the SAT, which is used by many colleges in determining whom to accept). This accomplishment required a great deal of work along the way, and it has been worth every bit of it.

By the time Annie entered middle school, I was equipped with a new Ph.D. in reading and cognition and had become a full-time member of the faculty at Denison University. From this vantage point I was able to look back on Annie's fairly normal acquisition of reading and writing processes. The ease with which she learned to read and write and the many ways that reading helped her speak and listen better led me to ask whether other children with prelingual deafness (the loss of hearing before learning language) who were taught their family's spoken language through use of their residual hearing were making the same sort of progress. Had we just had some kind of great good luck? In other words, did other children brought up in the auditory-verbal approach have similar results? It is certainly the case that some people perform better at verbal tasks than others, yet I questioned the data that were being used to predict that almost all people who are deaf or hard of hearing would suffer from lesser achievement in this area.

Studying the Reading and Writing Achievement of Auditory-Verbal Learners

My first study of this question involved trying to locate as many children with hearing loss as possible who had been taught language and speech through the auditory-verbal approach (Robertson & Flexer, 1993). Carol Flexer of the University of Akron and I sought contact with the families of children in auditory-verbal programs by distributing questionnaires at the June 1989 meeting of Auditory-Verbal International, Inc., in Toronto, Canada, and by sending questionnaires to therapists we knew were working with the approach. We asked parents to describe their child's hearing history, school(s), extracurricular activity, and the quality of the contact they had with children with normal hearing. We also asked about what they had done about reading before their child went to school and whether their child liked to read. Finally, we asked for test scores from standardized reading tests and for some indication of how much the child read each week. Obviously, we were looking for ways to compare the reading development of the auditory-verbal children with the reading development of children with normal hearing.

We decided we would analyze only those returned surveys describing school age children with prelingual hearing loss ranging from moderate to profound. We received completed surveys describing 54 such children in the United States and Canada and 29 such children in Switzerland and Germany. Of the North American children, the age range was 6 to 19 years, and 81% of them had a severe-to-profound or profound hearing loss. Roughly half were female and half male, and they lived in all regions of the United States and in the Toronto area of Canada. All but one of the children attended schools where they were placed in classes with children with normal hearing. Forty-four had always been placed in classes with children with normal hearing (fully mainstreamed); nine had been put in special programs where they were taught separately for part of the day, and one had been in a special "pullout" program throughout his school years. Twenty-four of the Swiss and German children had profound deafness, and all 29 of the total number were in schools with hearing peers.

The parents of all but one of the total number of 83 children described them as having daily contacts with hearing children, as being actively involved in extra-curricular activities, and as getting along well in the hearing world.

We received standardized reading test scores on tests created for students with normal hearing for 37 North American children and found that the average of the scores was at the 60.6th percentile rank. (A percentile rank score indicates that the test-taker scored higher than that percentage of the students on whom the test was normed. Test-makers select a representative group, test them, and then use their scores as benchmarks for comparison. Note that a percentile rank of 50 is an exactly average score because it signifies that the score is higher than the score earned by 50 percent of the original test-takers. A score at the 50th percentile on a test designed for the grade the child is in translates into reading exactly at grade level.) Of the 37 scores, 7 were below the 50th percentile, 14 clustered around the 50th percentile, and 16 were above the 50th percentile, suggesting that, in general, this group of students was doing better on reading tests than children with normal hearing. The Swiss and German parents were not able to send us standardized reading test scores because such tests are not in widespread use in those countries, but the 20 parents of children older than 7 reported that their children read as well as or better than the children with normal hearing in their classes.

Parents' reports for North American, Swiss, and German children told us that all but 3 of the 83 children had been read to by adults or others daily during their early childhood years. For the North American children, the average age for beginning to read was 5.3 years, with the earliest reader starting at 3 years old and the latest at 10 years old; all but 2 were beginning to read by age 7. In general, parents in all four countries described their children as liking to read, as reading beyond their school work, and as average to above average readers in comparison to the children they knew with normal hearing.

The results of this study are encouraging because they demonstrate that reading achievement comparable to that of children with normal hearing is possible for children with prelingual hearing loss, even if their loss is severe or profound. The children reported on are growing up in many parts of the world, and so it is neither the work of one talented therapist nor some kind of unusual, localized circumstance that is producing these results. Two factors stand out in the backgrounds of the 83 children: nearly all of them were read to daily from an early age and nearly all of them attend school with peers who have normal hearing.

Taking Another Look at the Reading and Writing Achievement of Auditory-Verbal Learners

Not long after the completion of the first study, I began another (Robertson, under review). This time I decided to visit three centers which had used the auditory-verbal approach for at least 20 years: Easton, Pennsylvania; Toronto, Canada; and Denver, Colorado. I was interested in gathering data that would provide a picture of the reading as well as the writing development and achievement of as many children and adolescents as possible who met the following criteria: (1) prelingual severe or profound hearing loss; (2) enrollment in public or private school from preschool on with peers with normal hearing; and (3) no other problem such as visual impairment, learning disability, or developmental delay.

Among the 38 children studied, unaided pure tone averages were distributed as follows: 11 had a 100+ dB loss, 10 had a 90–99 dB loss, 8 had an 80–89 dB loss, 6 had a 70–79 dB loss, and 3 had a 60–69 dB loss. All had been diagnosed by the age of 36 months, their time of beginning to wear hearing aids ranged from 2 to 42 months, and the onset of their auditory-verbal therapy was from 5 to 48 months.

Wanting to compare their vocabulary and comprehension achievement with that of children with normal hearing, I administered the Gates-MacGinitie Reading Tests to each child (the U.S. and Canadian versions for U.S. and Canadian children, respectively), and I asked each child in fourth grade and older to produce a short writing sample. The Gates-MacGinitie tests were designed for hearing children and "normed" on hearing children, meaning that the scores of thousands of hearing children provided the original "benchmark" performances on the tests. The original scores were analyzed statistically and distributed across the normal curve. When any child takes the test, the score he or she receives is based on a comparison between her or his responses and the responses of the children who took the test originally. By giving the Gates-MacGinitie test to children who are deaf or hard of hearing, I was able, then, to compare their reading achievement (as measured by that test) with the reading achievement of children with normal hearing.

To evaluate the writing samples, I arranged for regular classroom teachers in a large school district near where I live to read and score the samples. I did not tell them they were reading the writing of children who are deaf or hard of hearing; I only asked them to decide how each paper stood in relation to a performance scale they had been using for several years when they evaluated the writing of hearing children. I will discuss the results of these writing samples in Chapter Five.

I was also interested in trying to discover whether there were any particular factors that were associated with good reading achievement, and so I asked for information about when each child's hearing loss was diagnosed, the degree of the hearing loss, the age when hearing aids were first used, and how often and how long the child had had auditory-verbal or other therapy. In addition, I gathered data on whether and how the child had been read to before reading instruction began, whether the child was in a special class at school or mainstreamed into classes with children with normal hearing, and the financial status of the family.

An exhaustive search turned up 38 children who met the conditions outlined above (severe or profound hearing loss before language was learned, attendance at school with children with normal hearing, and the absence of learning disability, significant visual impairment, and developmental delay). Eight of the children had been in the first study.

The 38 children and adolescents were spread through school from preschool to university. All but 11 of the children attended school with children their own age. These 11 were one year older than their average classmate, their parents having decided to delay their beginning kindergarten or first grade. None had failed a grade and had to repeat it.

The results were in line with the parent reports of the first study. The average vocabulary score was at the 55th percentile and the average comprehension score was at the 57th percentile. Scores ranged from the 1st percentile to the highest possible, the 99th. Overall, the standardized reading test results were quite similar in their spread to standardized reading test scores for children with normal hearing, though the elementary, high school, and university students earned higher scores than did the middle school students. In their analysis of the writing samples, teachers experienced in evaluating the writing of children with normal hearing found only three of the papers to be unacceptable for their grade level. Although not every child and adolescent who was deaf or hard of hearing achieved an above-average score in reading and writing, we must keep in mind that because of the way standardized tests are formulated, half of any group tested — with normal hearing or not — will have scores that are below average in relation to the group's scores and half will score above average. Of importance in considering the scores of these readers and writers who are deaf or hard of hearing is that as a group they do not stand out as significantly different from readers and writers who have the advantage of normal hearing. This adds to our confidence that children who are deaf or hard of hearing can achieve reading and writing levels comparable to those of their hearing peers. I will revisit this study and its implications in chapters four and five, which deal with how children learn reading and writing.

Of further interest is that in a statistical analysis which looked for pairings of factors that were associated with reading and writing achievement, or the lack of it, only one pairing came out as important. Age of diagnosis, degree of hearing loss, age when hearing aids were first worn, the amount and frequency of auditory-verbal or other therapy, reading to the child, school placement with children with normal hearing, and the financial status of the family are all important factors affecting the development of each child. Statistically, however, the only pairing of two factors that predicted higher achievement was that of degree of hearing loss and magnitude of income. The lesser the impairment and the higher the income, the higher the reading and writing achievement. It is easy to see that the child with a severe loss quite likely has an easier time using the hearing that he or she does have compared to the child with a profound loss and so might learn language more easily. It is also easy to see that if a family has a higher income, it has more resources to use in paying for therapy, hearing aids, and learning experiences for the child. Parents in such families are likely to have more education and access to people who can help them than parents in less affluent situations. This is no different from the hearing world in which children of more affluent families score higher on standardized tests than children of poorer families (Kozol, 1985). It is not that children from affluent families are more intelligent in general than children from poorer families; it is that they have more, and richer, learning opportunities. This pairing of factors, then, is not surprising. What is surprising is that not one of the seven factors on its own predicted success or failure in reading and writing for the child who is deaf or hard of hearing.

An Outcome Study of Auditory-Verbal Graduates

Additional documentation of the success of children who learn how to listen to and use spoken language comes from a study of auditory-verbal graduates done by Goldberg and Flexer (1993). They surveyed people age 18 and older who had been students of therapists who had used auditory-verbal methods. Of 152 respondents, 86.2% had been fully mainstreamed in high schools with students with normal hearing, 151 had completed high school, and one had earned a G.E.D. (high school equivalency degree). More than 95% went on to some sort of post-secondary education, with 124 attending college or university. All but 15 of the college/university students were attending or had attended institutions that were not designed especially for students who are deaf or hard of hearing. While Goldberg and Flexer did not ask specifically about reading and writing achievement levels, at least average achievement compared to peers with normal hearing can be inferred for most of the respondents, given their educational accomplishments.

Evidence from the Mid-1950s

Only after completing my two studies, did I read that Daniel Ling had worked with 6- to 12-year-old children in Reading, England, in the mid-1950s and found good academic progress to be possible. In his words:

> *Standardized tests of reading, math, and spelling confirmed that most of the children were rapidly closing the educational gap between themselves and their normally hearing peers. After a few years, most, with continuing support from a visiting specialist teacher, successfully followed academic subjects alongside hearing children of the same age. Friendships with such children, formed in the classes they shared and during play breaks, led to extensive social relationships and conformity with behaviors observed among children at large. The children's speech and language skills increased rapidly to meet the standards of communication required to function effectively at home and in school* (Ling, 1993, p. 190).

Ling continues by saying that follow-up studies of children who were in his programs later in Canada show that many are bilingual in English and French, some have completed university educations, some have entered professional fields, and most have entered the hearing world with success.

Taken together, these reports suggest that reading and writing achievement comparable to that of people with normal hearing is possible for the child who has a hearing loss. It is the purpose of this book to describe one way of working toward that goal.

The Oral vs. Signing vs. Total Communication vs. Aural Debate

Because I have asserted thus far the importance of learning to speak the language spoken in one's environment in order to learn to read and write, I must make clear why that is so. It is simply this: In order to learn to read and write, the learner must know the spoken version of the language that is to be read and written. Further, the language the learner knows must have a version that can be written down. This may seem obvious, but it demonstrates in part why people who know only sign language do not ordinarily make great progress in learning to read English. In the next chapter I will discuss this at greater length. At this point, it is important to know something about the history of the education of the deaf in the United States so as to have a context for considering the various methods in the field.

The learning of language, *how* the language is best learned, and *which* language is to be learned have been major issues in the education of people who are deaf or hard of hearing in the United States for well over 150 years. Some have termed the controversy that has emerged pitting speaking (the oral approach) against signing (the *manual* approach) "The Hundred Years War," (Lou, 1988, p. 95) because each side has been so passionately defended by its proponents. Both methods of communication have long histories for people who are deaf or hard of hearing. Except where I note otherwise, the following is drawn from a history written by M.S. Lou (1988).

SIGN LANGUAGES

According to Lou, American Sign Language (ASL) and other manual approaches were used to the exclusion of others from 1817 through 1860, heavily influenced by Thomas Gallaudet's learning of a manual method from the French. Ironically, Gallaudet had sought to learn both methods but was turned down by the Braidwood family in England as a candidate for learning its oral method, a rejection that was to have an enormous impact on the education of those who have been and are deaf or hard of hearing in the United States (Meadow, 1980). In 1835, in the United States, public schooling for the deaf was separate from schooling for the hearing and was usually residential. Such schooling employed manual methods exclusively, and teachers of the deaf were expected to know and use ASL. But the oral approach was soon to be explored.

THE ORAL APPROACH

In 1844, Horace Mann, who is mainly remembered as the architect of the American common school that established the basic framework of public education in the United States, returned from Germany and the United Kingdom much impressed with the oral methods he had observed in those countries. His reports led others to make observational visits. While not all observers agreed about how successful the oral methods were, Mann's views were influential, and some schools began — with mixed success — to offer articulation training to their students who had some residual hearing. The Clarke School in Massachusetts and the Lexington School in New York were established as oral-only schools in 1867 and the first oral day school, Horace Mann School, was established in Boston in 1869.

A "COMBINED METHOD"

About this time, Edward Miner Gallaudet, the son of Thomas Gallaudet, decided that the deaf should learn signing as well as articulation and lipreading and urged this combination on the principals of the manual schools. Taking the position that each child's education should be developed according to his or her individual potential, Gallaudet championed the "combined method" in which both signing and speech were to be learned, though not in order to use them at the same time.

THE ORAL APPROACH BECOMES DOMINANT

During the 1880s, the oral approach became the dominant approach, mainly because of the influence of Mann, of Alexander Graham Bell, and of the pro-oral position taken by educators of the deaf in Europe. Bell used his father's Visible Speech approach and argued for keeping those who were deaf in the mainstream culture.

Lou (1988) comments on the education of the teachers of the deaf as being less rigorous as the century proceeded. At the time when the manual method was used predominantly, teachers were mainly young men with college degrees who added signing to their own considerable language skills. With the rise of the common school, education became more widespread for all (hearing) children, and teachers were in great demand; it was discovered that two women could be hired for the cost of one man, and as schools became more standardized, less educational background was required of teachers (Clifford, 1989, 307-308). The oral approach was on the rise at the same time, and teachers of the deaf were affected in the same way. Programs were established to train less well-educated young women to teach articulation and lipreading. The effects on deaf students of being taught by teachers with incomplete educations themselves are incalculable.

AN AURAL METHOD EMERGES

Oral methods were emphasized in most programs, then, from 1900 until 1960, though it is clear that some signing was allowed from program to program, particularly for those who could not master oral methods. As the development of hearing aids made the oral method look even more possible, some teachers and therapists began to focus on helping children learn to use their amplified hearing to the greatest extent possible. Max Goldstein of the Central Institute for the Deaf (CID) in 1914 developed what he called the "acoustic method" (Lou, 1988); Helen Beebe began developing what she called the "unisensory approach" in 1944 (Beebe, 1976); Doreen Pollack developed "acoupedics" during the late 1940s in New York, later moving it to Colorado (Pollack, 1993); and D. Fry and Edith Whetnall in England developed the "auditory approach" in the early 1950's (Fry, 1966). According to Daniel Ling (1993), a pioneer himself who worked from the early 1950's in England and Canada, there were early advocates of the approach in The Netherlands and Sweden, as well, all of them influenced by the early work of Urbantschitsch of Vienna published in 1895. Interestingly, the history of the concept of "improving the auditory capacity in deaf persons through conveying sound to their ears" can be traced back to the first century. Archigenes, a Syrian doctor who practiced in Rome sometime in the first century, attempted to bring sounds to deaf ears through a tube held up to the ear. He was followed by a long line of people who realized that many with deafness had residual hearing that could be used to help them learn to speak (Wedenberg, 1951, pp. 14-30).

But these approaches were not spread widely; they were not adopted by schools for the deaf, and their students attended schools for children with normal hearing which probably explains why these approaches did not receive a great deal of attention.

THE "TOTAL APPROACH"

By the 1960s, it was more broadly noticed that most people who were deaf or hard of hearing were, as we have seen, not making much progress in attaining age-appropriate achievement in school. The publication of *Sign Language*

Structure: An Outline of the Visual Communication Systems of the American Deaf (Stokoe, 1960) which legitimated sign language as a language, and the rise of claims for equality and equity for all marginal people during the Civil Rights movement influenced a swing back toward signing. The time was ripe for adopting "The Total Approach" developed by Dorothy Shifflet in the early 1960's for high school students and renamed "Total Communication" by Roy Holcomb in 1968 for use with elementary children. By 1976, "Total Communication" was defined officially by the Conference of Executives of American Schools for the Deaf as "a philosophy incorporating the appropriate aural, manual, and oral modes of communication in order to ensure effective communication with and among hearing impaired persons" (Garretson, 1976, p. 300, as cited in Lou, 1988). Meadows (1980) documents the lack of agreement about how Total Communication is to be implemented (Are signs and speech used simultaneously? Which sign language?) and asserts that the meaning of "Total Communication" changes depending on who is using the term, which makes it difficult to evaluate. In Lou's estimation, at the time of its proposal, Total Communication represented something of a truce in the "Hundred Years' War" in that all modes of communication were to be used with each person in the combination best suited to him or her, but she goes on to write, "unfortunately, this position was compromised and misinterpreted as it was translated in practice to mean simultaneous communication for all. In this form, it is now viewed by many as just a third camp in an expanded war between oral and manual approaches, and between English and ASL forces" (Lou, 1988, p. 95).

The Auditory-Verbal Approach

Little-noticed during the rise of Total Communication was the development of what is now termed the "Auditory-Verbal Approach." Helen Beebe (1976), Doreen Pollack (1985), Daniel Ling (1989), and others continued their work independently and quietly, not even meeting each other until 1972 at the first Auditory Conference in Pasadena, California. Initially, the organization they began was part of the Alexander Graham Bell Association for the Deaf and was called the International Committee on Auditory-Verbal Communication, the term "auditory-verbal" having been suggested by Ling. In the 1980s, it became the independent organization now known as Auditory-Verbal International. The approach emphasizes the intentional and careful creation of a language-rich environment in the home and in the school, coupled with intensive individual speech and language therapy from the earliest age possible. The goal is for parents, therapists, and teachers to help the child to use whatever residual hearing he or she has, amplified by the best possible hearing technology, so that he or she can acquire listening and speaking abilities as normally as possible. To make this happen, parents and others around the child must make use of every opportunity for listening and speaking in order to help the child learn more about listening and speaking. Language learning must go on all the time, not just in sessions with a therapist or teacher. Such learning is the same kind of learning that a child with normal hearing does "casually"; for the child who is deaf or hard of hearing, others must make sure that he or she is presented with all the sounds possible, both speech and environmental sounds. This is not as hard to do as it may sound at first. In later chapters, I will describe ways we did it.

Table 1.1. Auditory-Verbal Principles

1. Supporting and promoting programs for the early detection and identification of hearing impairment and the auditory management of infants, toddlers, and children so identified.

2. Providing the earliest and most appropriate use of medical and amplification technology to achieve the maximum benefits available.

3. Instructing primary caregivers in ways to provide maximal acoustic stimulation within meaningful contexts, and supporting the developing of the most favorable auditory learning environments for the acquisition of spoken language.

4. Seeking to integrate listening into the child's total personality in response to the environment.

5. Supporting the view that communication is a social act, and seeking to improve spoken communication interaction within the typical social dyad of infant/child with hearing impairment and primary caregiver(s), including the use of the parents as primary models for spoken language development, and implementing one-to-one teaching.

6. Seeking to establish the child's integrated auditory system for the self-monitoring of emerging speech.

7. Using natural sequential patterns of auditory, perceptual, linguistic, and cognitive stimulation to encourage the emergence of listening, speech, and language abilities.

8. Making ongoing evaluation and prognosis of the development of listening skills an integral part of the (re)habilitative process.

9. Supporting the concepts of mainstreaming and integration of children with hearing impairments into regular education classes with appropriate support services and to the fullest extent possible.

(Auditory-Verbal International, 1991, pp. 11-12)

Learning to Listen to a Spoken Language is the Key

Auditory-Verbal Principles are provided in Table 1.1 A close inspection of the principles demonstrates the hugely important role that learning to listen plays in the auditory-verbal child's life. It is precisely this listening that fosters the emergence and development of literacy. At this point, I want to make an important distinction. Children can learn non-spoken languages, and they will be able to communicate well using them. Each sign language is an intact, useful, and beautiful language that follows well-established grammatical rules. But, if children learn a sign language as their primary mode of communication, there is a good possibility they will not learn to read and write English (or whatever spoken and written language is used in their cultural location), for they will not learn enough about that spoken and written language to be able to use it for reading and writing. They will know a different language entirely, a language that is not written down to be read, but that is read as it is being produced. I am aware that sign language proponents argue that signing functions as a first language that will facilitate the acquisition of a second (spoken) language (King & Quigley, 1985). If this is so for children who are deaf or hard of hearing learning signing before learning a spoken language, then their reading achievement should be much greater than reports indicate. Perhaps the second language does not receive enough attention; perhaps there are fundamental differences in the processing of signs and spoken languages. More research is needed.

In the next chapter, I will discuss why knowledge of the language to be read is crucial to the development of reading and writing abilities.

2
What Is Known Currently About How Reading and Writing Work?

Highlights

▼ Reading and writing are extensions of listening and speaking.

▼ Knowing how to listen and speak precede learning how to read and write.

▼ Reading involves a complex interaction of knowledge of letters, words, and ability to use language.

▼ Good readers are both seeking and creating meaning as they read.

▼ Good writers are creating meaning as they write.

▼ Comprehension in reading and meaning-making in writing are dependent on language knowledge.

AT LEAST THREE BASIC WAYS OF EXPLAINING THE PROCESS OF READING AS DONE BY people with normal hearing have been developed. Whether one decides that one or the other of them is the most useful for understanding reading may not be as important as the fact that all of them require that the person doing the reading know the language that is being read. In this chapter, I will discuss these basic ways of explaining reading, detailing how they have been useful to me in forming my present understanding of how children who are deaf or hard of hearing learn to read if they have acquired language through the auditory-verbal approach, either through using their amplified residual hearing or the hearing they have gained through a cochlear implant.

Theorizing About Reading: A Letter- and Word-Based Approach

PHONICS

The first basic way of explaining reading is that the reader looks at the ink on the page and makes sense of it one letter at a time, "sounding out" each word, "hearing" the resulting word in her or his "mind's ear," and then upon hearing it coming to a recognition of what it is and what it means. This is the basis of what is known as the "phonics approach" in teaching reading. When this approach is used, the child is first taught to discriminate among various shapes, pictures, and objects. Some proponents of this method stress learning the concepts of *different* and *same* as grounding for learning to recognize the individual letters, their names, and their various sounds (Duffy & Sherman, 1972). As systematic progress with individual sounds is made, the child is introduced in an equally systematic way to letter combinations that occur frequently such as *sh, th, br, str,* and so on. Attention is paid to the child's ability to reproduce patterns of sound and attach certain sounds to certain patterns. To develop memory for the visual forms of pictures, shapes, and letters, games are played such as Memory (or Concentration) where pairs of cards are placed face down in random order and the players must discover pairings by alternately turning over cards one at a time until a match can be made from memory.

Reading books have been developed that contain vocabularies limited in prescribed ways so that the beginner will not have to encounter too many unfamiliar words. Schoolbooks such as these are called basal readers; in their use both teachers and students are taken step-by-step through the process of adding continuously to the new reader's repertoire of recognizable sounds, word parts, and words. The early Dr. Seuss books such as *The Cat in the Hat* work from this principle. In this view reading is a skill to be developed one step at a time. The task is envisioned as a decoding process in which each word is changed from print into sound. An easy way to think about this is that each letter signifies a sound, and the sounds are put together in left to right sequence in much the same way a computer voice synthesizer can "read" words into sounds.

PHONEMIC AWARENESS

Recently, researchers have begun to investigate a concept called "phonemic awareness" as a prerequisite for understanding the relationship between sounds and letters (see, for example, Adams, 1991; Griffith & Olson, 1992; Walser, 1998; and Yopp, 1992). A phoneme is "one of the set of the smallest units of speech, as the *m* of *mat* and the *b* of *bat* in English, that distinguish one utterance or word from another in a given language" (The American Heritage Dictionary, 1985, p. 932). Phonemic awareness is the ability to think about the sounds of language aside from thinking about the meaning of language (Griffith & Olson, 1992). It is a complex skill because the sounds in words change according to the sounds that accompany them; for example, identifying an *a* sound in *have* and an a sound in mark is difficult, because these two a's do not sound very much alike because of the letters around them.

The easiest tasks of differentiation are those found in rhyming words (Adams, 1990). In *mat* and *bat*, for example, the *m*, *b*, and *t* do not make much difference for the way we hear the *a*. Phonemic awareness is a prerequisite for understanding phonics, for understanding that certain sounds and combinations of sounds have specific letters and combinations of letters that are ordinarily associated with them (Griffith and Olson, 1992, p. 519; Juel, Griffith, & Gough, 1986). Some children with normal hearing and many children who are deaf or hard of hearing have a great deal of difficulty coming to this important insight that the words heard are made up of little bits of sound (Griffith and Olson, 1992, p. 516) According to Yopp (1992, p. 699), "It is the breaking down and manipulation of *spoken* language that is of interest." This understanding provides us with one rationale for the necessity of children learning the language spoken around them as preparation for learning to read that language.

SIGHT WORDS

Now, one can observe that not all words can be "sounded out" according to regular rules of phonics. For example, *take, rake, bake,* and *make* all follow the general rule that in a CVCe (consonant, vowel, consonant, e) word, the first vowel (a in this case) "sounds like its name" and the e is not pronounced ("silent e"). *Save* and *rave* behave in the same way — but what about *have?* As Smith (1978, p. 140) points out, the sound-to-symbol relationship of spoken and written English is exceedingly complex. In a study of 6000 words commonly found in children's reading books, 211 sound-to-symbol relationships were found, including *79 ways to pronounce a, e, i, o, and u.*

The sight word, or see and say, approach was designed to take care of the many irregularities in the English language. In this approach, certain sight words are introduced at specific times, again so that the new reader is not overwhelmed by too much unfamiliarity. The teacher might introduce the new reader to a list of words and even require some practice or drill with them before he or she is to read a story containing them. The object of this approach is to instill each word into the reader's memory so that it can be activated in its entirety when encountered on the page, without having to take time to "sound it out" and decide on a corrected pronunciation due to its phonic irregularities.

Both of these approaches are termed "bottom-up approaches" (Rumelhart, 1977, p. 128) because they both conceptualize the reader as being dependent on or driven by the text. In this explanation, the meaning is on the page, to be discovered by the reader. The question, "what does it mean?", implies that a meaning was put on paper by its author to be pried out by the reader by decoding the inky shapes (letters) into sounds and then putting the meanings of the individual words together.

PHONICS OR SIGHT WORDS?

There has been much argument over the years over whether a phonics or sight word approach is better for teaching children with normal hearing to read (see, for example, Smith, 1985, or Shannon, 1989). Reading lessons in most elementary schools rely heavily on textbooks and accompanying workbooks that make use of one or both of these approaches. Methods developed years ago are still in use, updated with "workbooks, worksheets, flash cards, games, puppets, computers, and floppy disks," and some assert that little has changed in reading instruction in most schools in seventy years (Shannon, 1989, p. xiv). There has been a concerted effort on the part of researchers and publishers to create materials that increase gradually in difficulty for teachers to follow step-by-step with the goal of producing good reading achievement. And yet, the phonics explanation of reading helps us only to a certain extent. It is interesting to note that Spanish-speaking children with normal hearing have difficulties similar to those of English-speaking children with normal hearing in learning to read Spanish, in spite of the regular and dependable letter-sound relationships in the Spanish language system (Ferreiro, 1990, p. 12).

Where have children who are deaf or hard of hearing been placed within the phonics vs. sight word controversy? In general, they have been assumed to be dependent on visual cues, "decipher[ing] the printed word using visual rather than phonological or auditory techniques" (Hart, 1978, pp. 6-7), and so the sight word approach has been tried more often with them.

Theorizing About Reading: A Context-Based Approach

As might be anticipated, the explanation that competes with the "bottom-up" explanation is called the "top-down" explanation (Rumelhart, 1977, p. 128). This view puts a more obvious emphasis on the language abilities of the reader, for every move the reader makes is interpreted as a language-based activity of one sort or another. In the "top-down" view, meaning is seen as residing in the reader's mind and memory rather than in the ink on the page as representative of the author's intention. The reader is seen as creating meaning during reading rather than identifying someone else's meaning. The reader is described as making a series of meaningful predictions on the basis of various aspects of the reading situation: the purpose the reader has for reading a particular piece; previous learning and background knowledge; the meaning the reader has created at any particular point in the reading; the context of the story and its similarity to other stories; the order of the words; the parts of speech of words; and the regularity/irregularity of spelling patterns.

An account of the process of reading developed by Kenneth Goodman and presented nearly 30 years ago in 1967 at the annual meeting of the American Educational Research Association (Marzano, p. 80) demonstrates a "top-down" view and describes the proficient reader as doing the following:

1. The reader works with each line of print from left to right, moving down the page, taking each line in order.

2. The reader selects particular print to stop and focus on briefly. Some of the focused-on print is in the center of her or his focus, and some is in soft focus. This allows the reader to think about single words and/or small groups of words.

3. The reader is guided by her or his knowledge of language and purpose for reading, the type of text being read, and her or his present understanding of the topic in order to locate cues that are useful in creating an understanding of what is being read.

4. Having done this, the reader assigns a guess or a tentative choice of meaning to the word or phrase.

5. Depending on the meaning he or she has already created, the reader decides whether what has just now been understood is reasonable.

6. If the guess is reasonable, the reader begins to expect the rest of the text to carry particular kinds of meaning. If the guess seems unreasonable, the reader must revise the guess and may reread portions of the text in order to do so.

7. The cycle continues.

In an approach derived from this explanation, stories for children to read are chosen because they connect in some important way to their experiences, so that it is easier for them to make sensible predictions. Letting children choose what they want to read about also leads to greater ease in predicting. Emphasis is often on having beginning readers tell their own stories to someone who puts them in writing. Then, with paper in hand, these early readers may read their own tales in their own words. In this way the stories and the words are highly predictable for the new reader, and he or she gradually acquires a repertoire of easily identified words and phrases.

Limitations of "Bottom-Up" and "Top-Down" Theories

There are some drawbacks to both of these explanations of reading. Instruction based on a "bottom-up" explanation may not focus sufficiently on meaning. Whether the beginning reader is being taught through phonics or sight words or a combination of the two, he or she may misunderstand the purpose of reading to be that of producing sounds that go with the shapes on the page. The processing of each word can become a tedious matter, so tedious in fact that the reader puts too much cognitive attention into the decoding of the shapes into sounds, and the result is simply making noises to go with symbols. Working memory can hold a limited amount of information for a limited span of time. "Sounding out" each word can result in working one's way through a sentence and arriving at the end only to have forgotten the words — and the meaning — decoded at the beginning (Smith, 1978, p 141). This reader is not bringing meaning to the process, creating meaning during the process, or taking any meaning away from the reading. Just as the computer does not comprehend what its own voice synthesizer says, the person who reads this way will have serious comprehension problems. It is possible for a person with little knowledge of a particular written language to be able to pronounce it from looking at the letters and word shapes, but still not comprehend it. If you have ever been in a country where a language other than your own is spoken, you might have experienced this phenomenon. Perhaps you began to catch on to the pronunciation rules so that you could put together a pronunciation of a word from its letters, but you still did not know what it meant. This can happen to the child who has normal hearing if he or she misunderstands the purpose of reading. This is necessarily part of the predicament the child (with normal *or* impaired hearing) is in who does not know the language that is to be read. The remedy that holds most promise, of course, is attending to the child's acquisition of the language that is to be read.

A potential drawback of the "top-down" explanation and the methods that grow out of it is that the reader could come to rely too much on guessing from the context what each word is, rather than establishing a dependable ability to recognize words by their letters or overall shapes. Confronted with a set of words in a new context, the reader might not be able to employ any workable word and letter-level strategies as helpful clues to what kind of words they are.

Theorizing About Reading: An Interactive Theory

Because of the overlapping drawbacks of "bottom-up" and "top-down" theories, interactive explanations of reading have emerged that describe mature readers as using information gained and created through both "top-down" and "bottom-up" means (see, for example, Rumelhart, 1985, pp. 722-750). Mature readers make use of multiple cueing systems and may appear to operate most often from a "top-down" direction, yet when meeting a strange new word or language with unusual word order, they will slow their reading to a crawl and make use of "top-down" contextual clues as well as the "bottom-up" strategies of looking for word parts to suggest meanings and for letters to suggest sounds. This interactive explanation holds that readers make flexible use of the many ways that decisions can be made about meaning during reading. The mature reader is so efficient in making these choices that during a particular reading event he or she can be unaware of even having made a processing choice while reading. It is also possible that the reader can use two or more ways of making meaning simultaneously (Bertelson, 1990, p. 94). Reading instruction that grows out of this interactive explanation attempts to help the learner make use of all the various processes involved in reading and does not focus on just one of them.

Theorizing About Writing

A PHONICS-BASED VIEW

Writing is the production side of reading and is clearly dependent on the writer creating a meaning and inscribing it somewhere so that someone — including the writer her or himself — can read it immediately or later. Explanations of writing processes mirror those describing the reading processes that I have discussed above. For example, writing has been conceived of as transcribing speech to paper in a reversal of the phonics explanation of reading. Techniques for teaching writing based on this view would begin with practice in forming the individual letters with the intent of progressing to drill in writing isolated words. The advice for spelling a particular word would be to "sound it out." Certain words would be taught according to a schedule that mirrors the level of reading of the child. This view carries with it some of the same limitations that phonics does (Britton, 1993, pp. 130-131).

A CONTEXT-BASED VIEW

Writing has also been described as representing thought in symbol (Ferreiro, 1991, p. 38). Teaching from this orientation would allow children to invent their own symbols, at least at the beginning of the process, and to request the spellings of words they want to know how to write.

AN INTERACTIVE VIEW

An explanation of how writing works based on a more interactive view holds that there is a rich interplay of all of the same systems that work in reading: word and letter sounds and meanings, word order and sentence structure, context and language conventions. Writers are seen as making use of all the various systems as they are needed in the meaning making process; at times two or more systems operate simultaneously, at other times the writer slows to focus on using just one of the systems.

Language Development and Reading and Writing

As I have already stated, acquisition of the language to be read is related integrally to acquisition of reading. The more complete the acquisition of the language is, the greater the reading achievement can be (Smith, 1978). Essentially, a person cannot read with comprehension that which is not already in her or his language repertoire. Most 5-year-olds with normal hearing are in control of all of the fundamental aspects of their language; they can construct appropriate sentences using conventional word order, and they can use all the parts of speech appropriately (Fry, 1966, p. 187). Articulation may or may not be mastered by this time, but articulation is not language, a point worth noting when thinking about children who are deaf or hard of hearing and their language development. Once language and reading are established to some degree, they can be used as vehicles for learning more language, but the essential work has by then been done, and the child then spends a lifetime building on this basic linguistic knowledge through an amassing of conceptual knowledge. New vocabulary representing new concepts enters the child's linguistic system as he or she finds it necessary to make new meanings. Concurrent with this development, many children with normal hearing learn to read simply by being read to with regularity (Durkin, 1966). They construct for themselves the relationship between what they hear and what they see on the page in relation to their own developing linguistic system, that is, by discovering patterns of words, letters, and ideas.

Children with normal hearing who grow up in environments in which people do not speak meaningfully to them and in which people do not expect meaningful responses from them are not likely to develop good language abilities or an adequate level of literacy (Britton, 1993; Heath, 1994). This information is crucial in thinking about and planning for the child who is deaf or hard of hearing, because it begins to explain why the more linguistic knowledge the child who is deaf or hard of hearing can accumulate, the better are his or her chances of learning to read well. Such learning can be predicted from the explanations of reading that I have presented, and so it is not surprising that Geers and Moog (1989) concluded as a result of their study of children who are deaf or hard of hearing who were taught through oral means:

> *The primary factors associated with the development of literacy in this orally educated sample are good use of residual hearing, early amplification and educational management, and—above all—oral English language ability, including vocabulary, syntax, and discourse skills* (Geers & Moog, 1989, p. 84).

Language, of course, is not simply a string of utterances that can be heard or read. As the child is figuring out the linguistic system, more is going on than the imitation of the speech of others. Children play with the structure of words and sentences and with thought itself as they begin to make meaningful sounds and put squiggles on paper. This play is their attempt to make sense of what they are experiencing, and it provides them a way to think about their experiences. Children experiment with word order, with vocabulary, with parts of speech, and so on, until they have created for themselves a linguistic system that works in their environment. In order to become literate, they must discover a system of writing that represents that which they are speaking and hearing.

READING AND WRITING ARE EXTENSIONS OF LISTENING AND SPEAKING

Reading and writing, then, are simply extensions of listening and speaking, and a good deal of listening and speaking must take place before reading and writing can begin to develop. This holds true for children with normal hearing as well as for children who are deaf or hard of hearing.

Listening and reading have much in common with one another. In both listening and reading, one must pay attention to another's words, make interpretations based on what one already knows, and construct a meaning for those words. Listening and reading might be called receptive activities because the impetus for them comes from outside oneself. Likewise, speaking and writing have similarities. In speaking and writing one must fashion a message for another, transferring thought to spoken or written symbol so that the other person can construct a meaning through encountering it. Speaking and writing can be called expressive activities.

SPOKEN AND WRITTEN LANGUAGE ARE DIFFERENT FROM EACH OTHER

An important difference exists, though, between spoken and written language. Each uses slightly different vocabulary, word order, and emphases. Spoken language does not have to supply the same amount of context as does written language. The speaker has the advantage, generally, of being able to receive feedback from the receiver of the message and so does not necessarily have to provide fully-formed or formal language. The topic of discussion may not even be named because the situation itself can make it apparent to the people who are talking. Written language, however, requires that the context be made explicit. The writer is responsible for trying to provide enough cues so that the reader can construct a suitable meaning and must follow agreed-upon conventions such as writing from left to right in rows of words from the top of the page to the bottom. Sentences must have predictable parts that appear in predictable and conventional orders: subject(s), verb(s), and, perhaps, object(s) with their appropriately placed modifiers. Because the reader is often reading a text in its author's absence, rules for using written language must be followed more carefully than rules for using spoken language in order to make text more dependable for its readers.

The Concept of Whole Language Instruction

Whole language instruction is an approach that is being used increasingly in elementary, middle, and high schools in the United States. Conceptually, it grows out of the interactive explanation of reading I dealt with earlier. The adjective "whole" in Whole Language means that language will not be carved up and examined in an artificial manner. Rather than concentrating on drills that isolate separate skills, learners are presented with whole and natural language as it is used for real purposes of communication. "Whole" also means that all aspects of language are used to get at meaning in the reading and writing process; contextual cues, sentence and story structure, and phonics and sight word emphases are all part of instruction, as they are needed to help the learner create meaning in relation to the words on the page.

In the words of Altwerger, Edelsky, and Flores (1987) as quoted in Kamii, Manning, and Manning (1991, p. 12):

> Whole Language is based on the following ideas: (a) language is for making meanings, for accomplishing purposes; (b) written language is language — thus, what is true for language in general is true for written language;

(c) the cueing systems of language (phonology in oral language, orthography in written language, morphology, syntax, semantics, pragmatics) are always simultaneously present and interacting in any instance of language use; (d) language use always occurs in a situation; (e) situations are critical to meaning–making.

WHOLE LANGUAGE IS AN APPROACH, NOT A METHOD

In using a whole language approach, the teacher does not follow a particular set of methods or method, but works from certain understandings and theories about language (Kamii, Manning, & Manning, 1991, p. 12). There are teachers who say they are using a whole language approach when they are not. For example, some misconstrue whole language as meaning that phonics will never be presented to learners in any form. In whole language, children will not be given drills on isolated phonics principles, but the sound-to-symbol relationships will be demonstrated and explained when doing so is helpful to the children in making meaning.

EXAMINING WHOLE LANGUAGE

(a) *Language is for making meanings, for accomplishing purposes* (Altwerger et al., 1987).

The whole language teacher will always use language in meaningful ways, whether in speaking/listening or in reading/writing situations. Children will have real opportunities to converse, read, and write about topics and experiences that are important to them in some way. In order to facilitate this, it is necessary that the teacher get to know the children in order to know what is going on in their lives. The children must be able to choose what they want to converse, read, and write about, and there must be purpose behind participating in these processes. For example, the birth of a new baby in a child's family would be a major topic of conversation. Conversation for a young learner might be about the baby's name, what the baby can do so far, and how the child is now a big sister or brother. Writing the baby's name and then reading it together would be an elementary step in the reading and writing process.

(b) *Written language is language — thus, what is true for language in general is true for written language* (Altwerger, et al., 1987).

Spoken and written language forms that are *in the same language* have a dependable relationship with one another. Whatever can be spoken can be written to represent exactly what was spoken; whatever can be written can be spoken with certain regularities, taking into account differences in pronunciation from one part of a country to another. These relationships can be discovered by the learner as he or she gains more facility with spoken language and encounters more written language. The dependable regularities make it possible for the learner to hypothesize about written language and to learn about it through testing the hypotheses and progressively revising them until a workable under-standing is achieved.

In translating from one language to another, though, there is not a one-to-one relationship between and among words and phrases. This would include signing in American Sign Language, for example; in translating to a spoken and/or written form of language, signed language must be interpreted, and so the translation into English will vary depending on the interpreter's word choices, just as would be the case in making the transition between English and French or English and Italian.

(c)   *The cueing systems of language (phonology in oral language, orthography in written language, morphology, syntax, semantics, pragmatics) are always simultaneously present and interacting in any instance of language use* (Altwerger, et al., 1987).

This statement comes out of the interaction explanation of reading dis-cussed earlier. As I have discussed above, when one uses language, whether it is written or spoken, many systems are interacting with one another. The language user can get the same information in a variety of ways, and the mature language user does so in the most efficient way possible, making strategic use of the interacting systems. For example, one might decide what the eighth word is in the following sentence on the basis of a variety of cues:

The family of Dashwood had been long *settled* in Sussex (Austen, 1811, 1992, p. 1).

The reader can make use of letter-sound relationships to read "settled" in this, the first sentence of Jane Austen's *Sense and Sensibility*. It has a regular letter-to-sound relationship. Bringing to the letters one's knowledge of the significance of "ed" as a past-tense ending aids in making sense of it. This comes under the heading of morphology which includes knowledge of inflection (in this case, the conjugation of verbs in particular tenses), derivation (the word's language origin), and formation of compounds. Knowledge of con-ventional word order, or the syntax, of the sentence helps, too. Even though the word order in this sentence is not usual for 20th centu-ry U.S. English, with a little experimentation and thought, it is apparent that a verb form is necessary in the place where "settled" appears. Knowledge of semantics, or meaning, provides another cue. A word such as "seated," which has letters similar to "settled," might be considered and then rejected as not fitting the conven-tional ways we use in English to talk about where people live, which brings us to pragmatics. Pragmatics considers the relationship between words and their users. It should be clear that there are many routes to making the meaning that the Dashwoods lived in Sussex for a long time; the reader does not need to travel all the routes in order to arrive at that meaning.

(d) Language use always occurs in a situation (Altwerger, et al., 1987).
Because language is used to communicate, it must always be about something. Presenting language without a situational context is presenting language that does not communicate. The language learner cannot learn anything new about language in this case and is merely manipulating letters and words without being able to decide on any meaning. As an example, this can happen with workbook pages where children are asked to match words that begin with the same sound when there is no meaningful context for the words themselves. Although this may not hurt the child, the same can be accomplished more efficiently by pointing out letter-to-sound similarities in words that he or she encounters in real stories.

(e) Situations are critical to meaning–making.
This statement follows from (d) above. Even mature readers need the context of a situation to make meaning of the letter and word shapes on the page. Knowing the second sentence of *Sense and Sensibility* will probably help you in constructing a satisfying meaning of the first sentence by adding to the context you have for the Dashwood family:

> *Their estate was large, and their residence was at Norland Park, in the centre of their property, where for many generations they had lived in so respectable a manner as to engage the general good opinion of their surrounding acquaintance* (Austen, 1811, 1992, p. 1).

My Present Understanding

I have come to see that children who are deaf or hard of hearing can and do learn the language spoken in their environment. Moreover, they learn all the various interacting processes within that language, and they use language to develop and to communicate their thoughts. Once they know the basics of the spoken language, they can begin to learn to read and to write it in order to augment it. Remarkably, their learning process is very similar to that of children with normal hearing. Listening plays a crucial role in the auditory-verbal child's life. It is precisely this listening that fosters the emergence and development of literacy.

In the next chapter, I will address why knowledge of the language to be read is crucial to the development of reading and writing abilities.

3 How Can My Child Learn Spoken Language?

Highlights

▼ With help, children who are deaf or hard of hearing can learn spoken language in very normal ways.

▼ Parents can help their children expand their language by asking them "why" and "how" questions.

▼ Creating and using language experience books is one way to help children learn language.

▼ Parents and others should read aloud to children from infancy.

▼ In order to help children develop language abilities, adults must talk with and listen to them as much as possible every day.

Language Development Is a Normal Process

LANGUAGE LEARNING FOR THE CHILD WHO IS DEAF OR HARD OF HEARING CAN follow the same patterns as language learning for the child with normal hearing. The difference is that the people around the child must take special care to make certain that it happens, and it will probably happen more slowly, mainly because sounds and language must be directed toward the child very intentionally and for a period of at least several years.

For the child with normal hearing, language learning takes place, barring any other disabilities, in a seemingly effortless way. One day the baby is babbling, and the next, it seems to the parent, he or she is putting together words and sentences! Of course it does not happen that fast; it's just that the parent of a child with normal hearing can afford to be preoccupied with other concerns and, therefore, does not see all the work the child does on her or his own to master language.

HOW CHILDREN WITH NORMAL HEARING LEARN LANGUAGE

Having made the claim that language learning for children who are deaf or hard of hearing follows the same general patterns that language learning for children with normal hearing does, I want to spend some time before moving on describing how children with normal hearing are thought to learn language.

First, it must be recognized that the role language plays in our lives is exceedingly important. We use language to represent our experiences and to make sense of them so that we can cope with them. To be sure, there are other ways to represent our experiences, but language is useful to us in bringing those ways together, as well (Britton, p. 19). The ability to put objects, actions, and attributes into categories and networks according to their similarities and lack of similarities underlies language. Until we can do that, we have no way of knowing what to expect, and we can make no predictions (Britton, p. 26). Luckily, the ability to categorize appears to be innate, and the child develops it by interacting with her or his environment (Pearson & Stephens, 1994, p. 25).

Many theorists regard language acquisition as filling a compelling social need in humans (Baron, 1995, p. 129-133; Vygotsky, 1962, p. 12; Britton, 1993, pp. 15-24). As the famous Helen Keller story tells us so dramatically, the discovery that "everything has a name" is a very exciting starting point that sets the stage for further discovery, and then all subsequent linguistic discovery is based on it (Britton, p. 36). While it may appear that children learning language are simply copying what they hear those around them saying, it is more complicated than that. Simply put, what children seem to imitate is "people's method for going about saying things" (Britton, p. 42). Children learning language spend a lot of time experimenting with sounds, with words and phrases, and with sentences, as they construct for themselves a communication system that meets their needs. This system must become conventional enough that those around them can understand it. The task of the language learner, then, is to discover and construct an understanding for her or himself of what people in their own environment are doing. While each child moves at an individual pace, the strategies that children use in learning language are surprisingly similar (Baron, p. 133). For example, many children as they discover the rule that in English one can combine "can" and "not" into "can't," "could" and "not" into "couldn't," and so forth will, through experimenting, combine "am" and "not" into "amn't," which, of course is not a word used conventionally. "Amn't" follows the rule, but is not used in English, and the fact that it is not used is part of what the child must discover. Brown and Bellugi's work has led them to the realization that it is not the parroting back of adult speech that leads to learning language; rather, "every child processes the speech to which he is exposed so as to induce from it a latent structure" (Britton, 1993, p. 46). The significance of the child producing "amn't" is that it demonstrates the child's understanding of the rule for putting two words together in a contraction. The child is producing meaningful speech that he or she has not heard others produce through discovering an underlying structure for the language to which he or she is exposed. It is this underlying structure that we spend our lives filling in with the content we call knowledge. One does not need to know how to talk about the underlying structure (the grammar) of her or his language in order to use the language used in one's environment. Learning the names of the parts of speech and how to identify them and learning rules that govern conventional word order can wait until much later; in fact, many people do not ever learn to talk about language in those ways. Learning language, then, is learning "how to do things with words" (Britton, 1993, p. 46), a creatively active process driven mainly by the language learner's curiosity and desire to make meaning.

There is considerable evidence that between the ages of two and four children are best able to acquire language (Meadow, 1980, p. 28; Britton, 1993, p. 95). If there is deprivation of some sort during and just beyond those years, the child will be likely to have life-long difficulties with language. It is as if there is a "window of opportunity" that, if missed, cannot be reclaimed with full adequacy. The child who is deaf or hard of hearing comes with the same "window of opportunity" as the child with normal hearing which explains the urgency of working toward developing language from the earliest possible age. I cannot stress enough the importance of providing the best amplification (hearing aids or a cochlear implant) and the richest language environment possible. When the "window of opportunity" closes at about age 4, the potential for learning spoken language is diminished severely, for the early years are so significant that they cannot be made up for later.

Language learning for the child with normal hearing begins with listening, though it is not just the listening that the child does that is important. The listening done by those around the child is equally important, for the responses the child gets help shape the language being learned. The responses the adult makes to the child's language are based on the adult's perception of the situation at hand. If the adult knows the child's experiences well, the adult can make responses that serve as explanations for the child's speech.

These explanations expand on the utterance of the child, and the child, in turn, has a chance to learn more about meaning–making through language. An example of such an expansion might go like this: the child says "Baby sleep," and the mother responds with "It's time for baby to be sleeping. Let's put Jamie down for his nap," if that is the case. In other instances, "Baby sleep" might elicit "Yes, the baby is sleeping. Jamie is very tired because we stayed out all morning," or "Are you ready to go to sleep?" The listening that is done by both the adult and the child is very important in establishing language in the child, for learning language and using language are dynamic, creative, and, above all, social processes (Britton, 1993, p. 49; Vygotsky, 1962, p. 51).

The Importance of the Parents' Attitude Toward Language Learning

Schlesinger (1988) has done some very interesting work in this area that demonstrates how parents' attitudes and approaches operate in the case of children who are deaf or hard of hearing. She studied a group of 20 preschoolers with normal hearing and a group of 40 preschoolers with profound hearing loss who had "no additional handicaps, had normal intellectual potential, and were from intact English-speaking families" (p. 265). She was most interested in the ways their mothers entered into talking with them. Observing that numerous researchers have pointed out that mothers deal with their children in at least two ways — either by trying to communicate or by trying to control — Schlesinger wanted to know the outcome of each style in terms of language achievement for children who are deaf or hard of hearing compared to children with normal hearing.

THE "ADVANTAGED PARENT"
Schlesinger makes a distinction between "advantaged" and "disadvantaged" parents. She labels parents who feel as though they have some control over their lives "advantaged," conceding that being in a relatively higher socioeconomic class has something to do with such advantage, but not defining such advantage as based solely on economic class. Factors such as more education, more books in the home, and a greater feeling of security also contribute to being "advantaged," explaining how a parent with a lower income could be regarded as "advantaged."

THE "DISADVANTAGED PARENT"
"Disadvantaged" parents, on the other hand, feel a comparative lack of control in their lives and may be in a lower socioeconomic class. They feel less able to ask questions of those working with their children and less capable of taking much initiative in the education of their children. While "advantaged" parents attempt to communicate with their children, "disadvantaged" parents tend to try to control their communication. Such control may show up in the form of the parent asking the child questions in a rote, routine way and expecting memorized, prescribed answers in return. It may manifest itself in the parent keeping conversation limited to the present or in the parent drilling the child constantly on letters, numbers, and colors. It is hypothesized that such attempts to control arise from feelings of powerlessness, of trying to gain some control where it feels as though there is little or none (Schlesinger, 1988, pp. 263-264).

This position of "disadvantage" is all too often where the parent of a child who is deaf or hard of hearing may feel he or she is, regardless of educational and socioeconomic attainment. According to Schlesinger, "many parents of deaf (and other disabled) children feel powerless because their children differ from them, because the future of their 'different' children looms uncertain in their minds, and because their usual parenting practices do not result in expected behaviors on the part of their children" (p. 263). In seeking an effective way to communicate with their children, they may respond to them in simplistic, all-or-nothing language. Yet this is not an issue of behavioral control for the children, but of language development. Just as the young language learner who hears normally needs enough space and freedom in a language-enriched environment to figure out how language works, so does the young language learner who is deaf or hard of hearing.

An environment in which an adult insists that the child repeat exactly what he or she says will only limit the child's language-learning opportunities. The controlling parent, whether the child has normal or impaired hearing, is attempting good-heartedly to program the child with useful information, but is missing the point that the child must construct an understanding of the world for her or himself. For children with normal hearing, language used to communicate generally produces the ability to use language to interact with and arrange their environment; language used to control results generally in the much less complex ability to describe what is occurring in the present, rather than to talk about what might occur in the future; to label things individually rather than being able to group things together into overarching categories; and to be less able to label feelings and other nonconcrete entities and attributes (Schlesinger, 1988, pages 264 and 268). Thus, linguistic deprivation can be the result of being in an overly controlled language environment for both hearing and deaf or hard of hearing children.

Parents' Dialogue Practices with Children

Schlesinger studied the mothers' dialogue practices with their children as toddlers and at ages 5, 8, and 16 years. She found that the encouragement of communication carried out through the "advantaged" style, especially in the early years, was associated with higher reading achievement in the adolescent years for both groups of children. The more the parents of the deaf children were able to overcome feelings of powerlessness, the more they were able to widen their interactions with their children. Such parents were able to help their children accomplish more than those who remained powerless in the face of their problems.

It is clear that the parent of the deaf child must get beyond questions such as:

"What is this?" and "What color is this?" which only require short, labeling responses and do not stimulate thinking and discovery of the properties of language. Parents and others in the child's environment need to be conscious about posing more complex "why" and "how" questions, and they need to follow them up with discussion and feedback to the child. The importance of this cannot be stressed enough; Schlesinger (1988) found that "those in our study who failed *why* questions at the age of 8 "failed" reading at adolescence" (p. 285). In thinking about why this might be so, it is helpful to revisit the explanation of the "top-down" view discussed in Chapter Five. Because meaning is created in the reader's mind and memory rather than residing in the ink on the page, the reader must have an ever-increasing store of meanings and representative words to rely on. Posing *why* and *how* questions contributes to that ever-increasing store and to the abilities necessary to increase it indefinitely.

SEEKING INTERACTIONS

Schlesinger (1988, p. 282) recommends that formal and informal work with the child should seek more active participation from the child and more interaction of ideas. Think about the last time you tried to learn to do something new. Perhaps someone showed you how to go "on-line" on a computer. If that person simply demonstrated the process to you, chances are you were not able to duplicate all the steps when you tried to perform them on your own. If, instead of being shown how to go "on-line," you were able to push the keys on the keyboard yourself, you were probably more able to carry out the process yourself when you were on your own. The difference is your level of participation. Watching someone else does not require you to participate and does not help you conceptualize the process; participating in the process itself is more likely to do so. It is the same for the language learner; active participation paves the way for more interaction of ideas, because the child can begin to tap into and try out her or his store of concepts and language for them. Bit by bit over time, interaction with the adult language user gives the child information about how to use the language.

USING ACTION AND CONCEPTUAL WORDS

Recalling that the overuse of naming words for objects ("What is this?"; "What color is this?") yields lower overall language achievement, it should be apparent that using more verbs and descriptive words to achieve more active language will augment the child's language (Schlesinger, 1988, p. 282). It should be easy to see that whatever can be said is far more interesting when action words and conceptual words are added to the conversation. Looking for examples in children's books is a good place to get some ideas for expanding on one's language with children. *Richard Scarry's Busiest People Ever* always delighted Annie. In one story about Mr. Frumble's bad day, Mr. Frumble *"forgot* to open the garage doors before he *backed* the car out (Scarry, p. 24)." "He *stopped* to *shop* at the supermarket" where he knocked over a stack of cans (Scarry, p. 24). "At the barber he *fidgets* so much that the barber *cuts* his necktie by mistake" (Scarry, p. 25). "Mr. Frumble how *did you get* your car on that new road? It's not ready yet for drivers. The workers are still busy *building* it (Scarry, p. 30).

Another book she liked, *Quick as a Cricket*, provides good examples of language which builds concepts: "I'm as quick as a cricket . . . I'm as slow as a snail . . . I'm as happy as a lark (Wood, 1982)." Building this kind of communication into daily talk draws the child into the process and allows her or him to conceptualize the language's structure through actually using the language.

Much of what is said to the child who is deaf or hard of hearing by the parent who feels powerless serves to keep the child in the present, preventing her or him from learning to speak about, and probably to think about, the future and the past. Schlesinger found that "the future is mentioned less frequently by disadvantaged and deaf children" (1988, p. 284), bringing the focus again to the role of the parent and the importance of the parent not feeling powerless.

TALKING *WITH* IS BETTER THAN TALKING *TO*

In order to draw the child in, one must talk *with* the child, always expecting a meaningful response, rather than talking *at* or *to* the child. Whoever (parent, sibling, teacher, therapist, etc.) knows a great deal about what the child has experienced is in a good position to make sense of the child's utterances. For example, I knew that Annie liked strawberries and that we had gone strawberry picking as a family, so when she talked about strawberry picking, I could understand her utterance even though she could not pronounce "strawberries" or "picking" clearly at a young age. I could use the conversation to enlarge on Annie's understanding and memory of what we had done and to pronounce both "strawberries" and "picking" clearly as a model for Annie. The interaction between the two or more participants makes the talking a conversation from which the child can learn, rather than a one-way recitation period during which the child is powerless and under the control of another who feels powerless. Turning yet again to Schlesinger: "Deaf children frequently are and see themselves under the control of others. They have been subjected to an excess of control talk from parents who have not themselves felt in control" (1988, p. 283). Concentrating on talking with the child gives everyone, child and parent (therapist, teacher) alike, more positive control.

The Auditory-Verbal Approach and Language Learning

Many who work with and write about literacy and deafness begin with the assumption I have been discussing that learning language is the basis for learning to read, but then they give up on the possibility of the child who is deaf or hard of hearing being able to learn the spoken language of the child's environment. It is easy to find such statements as these in the literature: "[T]he development of English is slow and difficult for deaf children. . . . It is unlikely that any typical deaf child ever acquires the necessary language base for reading before reading instruction begins" (King & Quigley, 1985, p. xiii). King and Quigley continue by saying that if the acquisition of language could be accomplished, then special approaches and materials for reading in the case of deaf children would not be needed. A main problem, they say, is that deaf children are having to learn a language and how to read it at the same time which overtaxes working memory and interferes with both processes (King & Quigley, 1985, p. 17). In their view, three remedies exist: (1) developing better speech in more children who are deaf, as Ling's work demonstrates is possible; (2) developing other means of teaching reading that do not depend on speech coding or recoding; and (3) finding other ways for those who are deaf to learn information (King & Quigley, 1985, p 23).

It is the first remedy that is the most promising. First, it has been demonstrated that it is possible for a significant number of children who are deaf or hard of hearing to learn to read and write well. In reading the recommendations of King and Quigley, I believe one must regard "speech" as implying "language" so as not to fall in the trap of concentrating on correct articulation at the expense of meaning–making. The second remedy ignores the integral relationship between spoken and written language. The third holds out the hope that information can be gained in a variety of ways. Of course this is true, but it is the ability to put such information into language that enables us to think and communicate about it. According to Britton (1993, p. 72), "We do not learn from the higgledy-piggledy of events as they strike the senses, but from the representation we make of them." A given event takes shape and is interpreted as we use language to talk about it (Britton, 1993, p. 30). There is no need to block out any of the many ways of taking in information, but to drop spoken and written language out as a main way of learning information is to leave the child who is deaf or hard of hearing without a major resource. To be successful in this regard, the family of the child who is deaf or hard of hearing must structure the environment so that it is friendly and supportive of language learning. Britton recognizes the need for the family to be adaptive to the language learning needs of the child with normal hearing:

> *Since it is by talking that a child learns to talk, the best way of helping him learn will take the form of fostering his explorations and his participation in family activities. One kind of fostering lies in the opening up of new fields — and the world to be explored through stories and books in general need not wait until he can read them for himself. Another kind of fostering lies in modifying the pattern of family activities in order to accommodate what he can contribute* (Britton, 1993, p. 94).

If even the families of children with normal hearing must modify their patterns in order to accommodate the child's needs, then so must families of children who are deaf or hard of hearing. The difference is that they must do so more intentionally.

LEARNING LANGUAGE THROUGH THE AUDITORY-VERBAL APPROACH

And so I turn to the auditory-verbal approach to the learning of language. The auditory-verbal approach enables the child who is deaf or hard of hearing to make use of the very natural process of learning language. Babbling develops in the child with normal or impaired hearing first as noises in response to both pleasant and unpleasant stimuli and continues as a pleasurable activity in itself. Babbling serves to help the child discover the possibilities for sounds and begins to establish an auditory feedback loop in the child with normal hearing (Fry, 1966, p. 188-189). This feedback loop serves as the foundation for learning to listen to and interpret speech and environmental sounds. For the child who is deaf or hard of hearing, there must be intervention for such a feedback loop to be established; the child needs to produce his or her own sounds and to hear his or her own sounds, as well as to hear the sounds of others so as to compare them with his or her own. The auditory feedback loop that is established helps the child learn to use the appropriate muscles for speech. Just as the child with normal hearing comes to use the sounds that he or she hears; so can the child who is deaf or hard of hearing (Fry, 1966, p. 190).

The necessary intervention for the feedback loop to develop involves the consistent wearing of two hearing aids or the use of a cochlear implant, bringing sounds to the attention of the child, and creating an environment that is rich in speech and language — the language-enriched environment of the "advantaged" family. As technology improves, it is becoming easier and easier to surround the child with usable and meaningful sound (Ling, 1989, p. viii). While some establish a cutoff point below which a child might be expected to learn the language spoken by those around him or her, it can be said more correctly that "the amount of speech a child develops depends not so much on the amount of hearing *per se* as upon the use he is able to make of his hearing for language-learning" (Fry, 1966, p. 201).

Two children with similar audiograms can turn out very differently in their ability to use speech and language; the one who is in the presence of early and repeated instances of meaningful speech and language can become the proficient language user while the other may have great difficulty in doing so. Note that I am being cautious in this claim. The child in the language-enriched environment *can* become a proficient language user. We must remind ourselves that children with normal hearing vary in their abilities to use language, and so will children who are deaf or hard of hearing. The point is to create the best environment possible for language development just as we would do for a child with normal hearing so that the child who is deaf or hard of hearing can make as much progress as possible.

Even given the best language-enriched environment possible, the linguistic progress of the auditory-verbal child will probably be slower than the progress of the child with normal hearing, but *there is every chance that the auditory-verbal child's speech and language will develop in very normal and predictable ways* (Fry, 1966, p. 204). This is the premise underlying the following chapters of this book.

Many excellent books exist which describe the auditory-verbal approach in great detail. Among them are: Ling, D. (1989), *Foundations of Spoken Language for Hearing-Impaired Children;* Ling, D., & Ling, A. (1978), *Aural Habilitation;* Estabrooks, W. (1994), *Auditory-Verbal Therapy for Parents and Professionals;* Vaughan, P. (Ed.) (1976), *Learning to Listen;* and Goldberg, D. (Ed.) (1993). Auditory-Verbal Philosophy: A Tutorial *(The Volta Review, 95).* Full citations for these are included in the references in the back of this book, and I urge you to make use of as many of them and others as you can.

Language Experience Books

The most useful tool for helping Annie develop language was the language experience book. Helen Beebe introduced us to its use the first time we met her, when Annie was $2^1/_2$ years old, and she called it simply an experience book. I recognized it as part of the language experience approach to the learning of reading (Durkin, 1993), about which I'll write more in chapter five and see it as the natural extension and record of the many ways that language comes into one's life. Thus I have added "language" to its title because "language" reminds us of our goal in using the book.

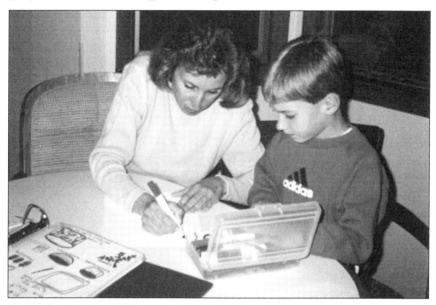

Figure 3.1. At this child's age, the adult and child take turns writing in the experience book and drawing pictures.

HOW-TO'S FOR THE LANGUAGE EXPERIENCE BOOK

The language experience book begins its life as a blank notebook or book of some sort. Into it go words, phrases, and sentences that have been an integral part of the child's experience in the very recent past. The words, phrases, and sentences are accompanied by a sketch drawn by someone, by a photograph, or by a picture cut out of a magazine or newspaper. Ideally, the words, phrases, sentences, and pictures come right out of the child's experience on the day they are added to the book; waiting too long makes them irrelevant. The person doing the book with the child (usually a parent, though it can be anyone who spends significant time with the child) must stay alert during the child's day to experiences that are meaningful to the child. This is very important. Children learn what interests them, what is important to them in some way (Smith, 1978), just as you probably do if you reflect on this point honestly. At the beginning, the parent chooses what to put in the book, mainly because at that point the child does not have enough language to communicate about what he or she wants to put in it. As time goes on, the child should be consulted about what he or she wants to put in the book. The parent can make judicious choices of words, phrases, and sentences based on what the child can say and understand already, always trying to stretch the child's vocabulary and usage. An easy way to view this is that the process is the same as the approach I discussed earlier in this chapter where the adult expands on the child's utterance, only in using the language experience book the language is recorded in writing and is represented by pictures so that it can be revisited. The language experience book can become a favorite story book that is read over and over again. As the child's knowledge of language grows, he or she can formulate more complicated words, phrases, and sentences to talk about the experiences in the book and so can the parent, teacher, or therapist, thus expanding on and stretching the child's language. The book is a tool for talking about (applying language to) the child's daily experiences and can be used very flexibly. Years later as I look back at Annie's books I see a rich record of her toddlerhood and early childhood, but that is not the point of the books at the time they are being used; it is simply a nice benefit to be enjoyed later.

It is important that the person making the book not be a perfectionist about it. The pictures need not be perfect, and the written language needs to be that which is used in the child's listening environment, not storybook language. The child must be allowed to pore over the book anytime he or she wants to do so, and there should be regular conversations with an adult about the pictures, using the language that is written with them as well as language that expands on what is written. The book serves to remind one what to talk about with the child, and having a book going at all times serves as a prompt to talk with the child regularly. Repetition through repeated use of the book gives the child many opportunities for practice and expansion.

A FEW EXAMPLES

In Figure 3.2, you can see an entry I made in Annie's book when she was about three and one-half. The main event of that day was going to story hour at the library, and so I added it to the book. I thought it was important to record it as though she was the one writing it because I hoped we would reach a time when she would be dictating to me what to write, and so it is written from her point of view. At that stage she was not able to put together sentences as complex as the ones in the entry. I was not sure that she even understood such sentences, but I knew she needed to be exposed to them. I also knew that it was quite possible that she had picked up little of the story that was read during the story hour. It was enough at that point to use language that named people in her life, to comment on the content of the story briefly, and to introduce one new word: *shape*. The simple drawing emphasizes features she was interested in at the time: eyelashes and her friend Molly's long hair. It gave us much to talk about on numerous occasions, it was interesting to her, and it provided a model of the kind of language that surrounded her, even though she could not always hear and process it.

3/19/81

Today Mommy took Molly and me to
the library to hear stories.
One story was about a bunny
who had to go to the hospital.

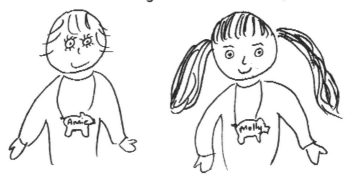

Our name tags are in the
shape of a pig.

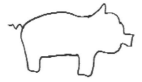

Figure 3.2. An example from Annie's language experience book.

I played on the swing. I was rolling around.

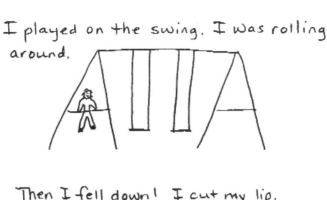

Then I fell down! I cut my lip. It started to bleed. I cried.

Mommy came to get me.

Daddy called the doctor. The doctor said, "OK, Annie" "Eat some popsicles."

Daddy went to the store and bought some popsicles.

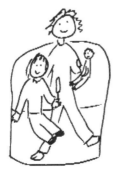

I sat on Mommy's lap and ate a popsicle.

I gave some to Mark, too.

That was Mark's first popsicle.

Figure 3.3. An example of a sequence of events depicted in Annie's language experience book.

Another way of constructing a language experience entry is to tell a story. In Figure 3.3 is an entry that describes the sequence of events that occurred when Annie fell from the swingset and cut her lip. Such a story provides a model for putting events in a conventional order so that the story can be related to another person. It also demonstrates how to tell someone what somebody else said, and it reinforces the concept "first" because Annie knew her baby brother had not had a popsicle before this day.

USES FOR THE LANGUAGE EXPERIENCE BOOK
The language experience book should be used to spark comfortable conversation about a concept or event. It can also be used to communicate to others about what is going on in the child's life. Taken to the weekly language and speech therapy session, it gives the therapist a sense of the child's interests and can serve as a catalyst for parent and therapist to make decisions together about what to emphasize. The book should not be used to present concepts to the child in a predetermined order or as material about which the child will be "quizzed." Its purpose is to present natural language in a meaningful context and to stimulate exchanges of language. In the next chapter, I will discuss how the language experience book can become an early reading book.

Reading Aloud to the Child

Numerous studies have shown that reading to children with normal hearing and surrounding them with print materials are both integral to their acquisition of reading (Durkin, 1966; Teale, 1978). In my own research I have found that children who are deaf or hard of hearing who read at average to above average levels have been read to from an early age (Robertson, 1993). Parents told me over and over again that they had read to their children on as close to a daily basis as they could manage. My own experience was that sitting Annie on my lap and holding a book together enabled me to speak directly into one of her hearing aid microphones as I read the book to her, thus creating a favorable sound-to-noise ratio and establishing a good listening environment. Reading together was a very pleasant activity that fostered an important closeness between us.

Reading aloud to a child does more than foster closeness. Through repetition with particular books, the child learns a great deal about language, especially about book language. The task of the child is to figure out how the language system works, and books provide a regular and dependable source of information that parallels that which the child is hearing on a daily basis. For example, the child learns about reading from left to right and top to bottom, about turning pages from right to left, about conventional and thus predictable word order, about using context by connecting words with pictures, and about sound-to-letter relationships.

Most important in reading to a very young child is to keep it fun for both the child and the adult. Allowing the child to choose which book to read helps her or him by ensuring that the book is interesting in at least some way and introducing new books as it feels right to do so can be fun for the adult. Many children will want to have the same book read over and over again, and that is a good practice. It is likely that children ask for the same story to be read over and over again until they have exhausted the questions they have about it (Lewis & Young, 1991). These are questions that the child most likely cannot articulate, but that have to do with relating the structure of language and the content of the story to her or his world.

Some children are not interested in the words on the page initially and are more drawn to looking at the pictures. There is no need to worry about this because connecting the spoken word to the pictures is an important part of language learning.

As reading progresses, some children enjoy having the adult point to the words as he or she reads. This is fine to do, but not necessary. It is important to relax and enjoy the story so that the child can discover the connections he or she is ready to make. Therefore, the reader should avoid turning these early reading sessions into instructional sessions. It may seem that the child is getting little or nothing from the reading, especially during the early phases when he or she may not be able to express much in spoken words. We can relax about this by reminding ourselves that children with normal hearing spend at least a year of life listening before beginning to speak. A child who is deaf or hard of hearing will need at least that long a period of listening after receiving ade-quate hearing aids, and reading to her or him becomes part of that listening. Further, as we consider reading an extension of listening and speaking, learn-ing to read will be possible after listening and speaking are established.

Parents often ask whether they should ask questions during and after the reading of a story. I would say yes if the questions come naturally out of the reading, or if the reader discovers somehow that the child has a fundamental misunderstanding of the story, but no, if the questions turn into a grilling of the child to see what he or she remembers. For example, at the end of *Little Red Riding Hood*, one might ask a child just beginning to learn language to point to a picture of Red Riding Hood doing different things in the story. ("Show me where Red Riding Hood is walking down the path"; "Show me where the wolf is running away") As language learning progresses, questions that generate discussion of the story are the best sort of questions to ask. For example, at the end of *Little Red Riding Hood*, one might ask, "What do you think Red Riding Hood did next?" or "What do you think Red Riding Hood learned?" These are questions that ask the child to think beyond the story, using the story and her or his imagination and feelings to think about the story. The asking of questions should develop into a two-way street, and so the child should be encouraged to ask questions of the adult, as well. The child's questions can give the adult insights into the meaning the child has created of the story, and can, in turn, prompt an explanation or the next question from the adult. Doing this, even in very simple fashion, becomes a model for the child of how people communicate with one another about something they both find interesting.

"READ IT AGAIN, MOMMY! READ IT AGAIN, DADDY!"

Keeping in mind that children usually request the same story again and again in order to learn something new each time (Lewis & Young, 1991), the adult reader can attempt to become aware of what the child is trying to learn each time and then use that information to make decisions about what to read or present next. Perhaps the child is focusing on the sequence of events in the story and is beginning to use words such as "before," "after," or "next." This might show up in the child's question "What did Red Riding Hood do before she went to Grandma's house?" The adult's next question might use "before" in it: "What did the wolf do before he went to Grandma's house?" Such a question provides an opportunity to see another example of the word being used. It also suggests that adding "after" to the talk would be a good next step.

Another reason children ask for the same story again and again is that they make some kind of emotional connection to it. These emotional connections are very important. Knowing some books as "old friends" stimulates wanting to discover other books that provide that kind of meaning in one's life. Children who grow to love books are very likely to become good readers.

Talk, Talk, Talk — In Meaningful Ways!

All through the life of any child, talking in meaningful ways is critical to her or his development. This is especially true for the child who is deaf or hard of hearing, because he or she misses significant portions of what people say. Consequently, this child needs many more representations of language than does the child with normal hearing. Parents, friends, teachers, and therapists, in short, everyone who comes into contact with the child who is deaf or hard of hearing should talk directly with the child as often as possible, wait for responses and respond to them. In auditory-verbal therapy, the therapist and the parent doing lessons concentrate on the child's learning to listen and so will usually cover their mouths while talking to the child. In day-to-day interaction, this is not necessary, though; establishing normal conversation habits is more important than testing the child constantly on listening. Paying attention to and working toward the optimum listening conditions in a house, store, or classroom and then talking with the child as one would talk with any child will enable the child to store up listening events that contribute to learning and using spoken language.

4
Can My Child Learn to Read in Natural Ways?

Highlights

▼ Even children who are deaf or hard of hearing can move smoothly from learning to talk to learning to read.

▼ Over a period of time, children construct knowledge about language, about the world around them, and about how to read a book.

▼ The parent of a preschool child should make sure the child has a rich amount of experience with books and people before beginning formal schooling.

▼ Everyday activities provide excellent opportunities to talk with children and to develop fluent language and a broad vocabulary.

▼ The language experience book can become a beginning reading book.

Reading Development Follows from Language Development

IN MOST CHILDREN WITH NORMAL HEARING, THE DEVELOPMENT OF LANGUAGE moves very naturally into the development of reading and writing, barring certain kinds of processing difficulties usually termed learning disabilities. The same can be true for children who is deaf or hard of hearing. I cannot stress enough the importance of working toward spoken language fluency and the intentional building of broad background knowledge with the child who is deaf or hard of hearing. Keep in mind that I am not urging perfect articulation or even particular attention to articulation, especially during the early stages, because being able to understand and construct one's own meanings is far more important than being able to speak clearly. Our own experience with Annie was that her articulation improved as a positive by-product as she began to see in print sounds that she ordinarily did not hear and so did not have the opportunity to pronounce in the early stages of language-learning.

Developing Background Knowledge is Essential

An important psychological theory called schema theory helps explain my insistence on developing language and content. Schema theory holds that each of us carries with us many, many overlapping and interconnected frameworks of all kinds of knowledge that we gain as we go through life (Anderson & Pearson, 1984). These frameworks are our background knowledge. Some knowledge is procedural; it helps us know what to do when. In reading, an example of procedural knowledge would be that in English we look at the words from left to right and at lines of words from top to bottom on the page. We also turn the pages so that we work through a book turning pages from right to left, right to left, over and over again until we come to the end. Another kind of knowledge is semantic; it tells us the conventional meaning to attach to words and phrases, that is, it tells us what the words and phrases mean to most people in our culture. An example of semantic knowledge can be found in words that carry more than one meaning. "Tear" can mean to rip something apart, or it can mean a drop of moisture coming from the eyes; it is the semantic context that makes the difference.

The broader and more complex the frameworks of knowledge are in the beginning reader, the more the beginning reader will be able to use her or his background knowledge to make sense of what is on the page. Being able to predict what word, kind of word, or idea might come next is very important in understanding what someone is saying to us in speech, as well as in words written on a page. It is this ever-growing network of interwoven bits of all types of knowledge that allows any one of us to come to reasonable and workable understandings.

With growth of background knowledge comes the ability to make inferences which are really just "educated guesses" or hunches about what will come next based on what has come before. Piaget's work in describing how children construct knowledge is very useful in understanding reading because it suggests that children do not just take knowledge in as a whole, but instead construct it over a period of time, seeking more (and more complex) understandings of the relationships between and among different items (Kamii, 1991). Children do a good deal of experimenting with knowledge, meanings, and words. While what they say and do may appear to be random, a great deal of it is driven by a quest for making meaning out of what is going on. For example, Piaget studied how boys thought a bicycle worked. At ages 4 to 5 and 5 to 6, the children in his study mentioned only the pedals and the wheels as making the bicycle work (Kamii, 1991, pp. 20-23). It was not until the age of 8 that most of the boys in his study were able to speak about the relationship between the rider, the pedals, the chain, the cog-wheel, and the wheels. With growth and maturity, a particular explanation is outgrown, and a new one, complete with new terminology, must be developed to take its place. This position about learning parallels the view taken by James Britton about language development described in Chapter Four, demonstrating the integral relationship between thought and language.

Creating a Rich Literacy Environment

In this chapter I will lay out some of the practices I have found to be useful in helping the preschool child who is deaf or hard of hearing to become ready to read. This can be done by creating a rich literacy environment so that the child can make important discoveries about language in its spoken and written forms. The practices I offer are meant to go along with speech and language therapy, such as auditory-verbal therapists provide, and are intended to prepare the child for entering kindergarten along with peers with normal hearing. While many children with normal hearing enter kindergarten already knowing how to read, many do not (Durkin, 1993, p. 75), and so the goal for the child who is deaf or hard of hearing does not have to be knowing how to read when entering kindergarten. The goal is to prepare the child so that he or she is ready for formal instruction, which usually comes not in kindergarten but in first grade. I also offer extensions of the practices so that support can be offered to the child as he or she matures.

I am starting from the premise that the child who is deaf or hard of hearing has the same challenge in most respects as the child with normal hearing in learning to read and write. The main difference is that the child who is deaf or hard of hearing must have an even richer literacy environment — in fact, the richest possible literacy environment — so that he or she has the optimal access to words, ideas, and well-formed language. A hearing child needs to hear a word or phrase in a meaningful context in order to assimilate it into his or her schematic network (Ling, 1978, pp. 44-45); the child who is deaf or hard of hearing must encounter it many, many times in a meaningful context because the quality of each encounter is in doubt, especially at the beginning when the child cannot speak enough to make clear what meaning he or she is constructing in the presence of particular words or phrases. For this reason, it is helpful to think of the child's needing to be inundated in language and meaning–making in both spoken and written forms.

I cannot stress enough how important it is to talk *with* the child as often as possible. Such talk must be meaningful and purposeful, and the adult must *listen* carefully to the child's utterances and try to make sense of them. Rather than listening for mistakes to correct, the adult should be listening for meanings to which to respond. I found that trying to correct Annie's pronunciation while putting off the meaning was ineffective, for doing so negated Annie's efforts to convey something to me. It is very hard to fight off that impulse to correct the articulation first, but it should be done because pronunciation is not language. Such corrections can be made later. Meaningful talk, sustained through childhood and into adolescence, provides an excellent way of helping the child increase language facility and fosters the even more important emotional connection between parent and child.

Knowing What Your Child Knows and Putting Language to Real Use

At least when the child is young, the parent knows the body of words that the child knows and knows the experiences he or she has had, which makes it easier to guess what the child is saying. This is true for children with normal hearing as well; the difference is that the child who is deaf or hard of hearing will probably be older when he or she is at the beginning stages of speaking, and the beginning stages will last longer.

In any case, the adult needs to be patient with the approximations of speaking (and later, reading and writing) that the child makes en route to mature uses of language.

The adult needs to create real reasons for listening, speaking, reading, writing, and thinking by including the child daily in activities that require listening, speaking, reading, writing, and thinking. Obviously, the ability of the child to enter into certain activities will be different at different ages and stages of development. The idea is to draw the child into an activity in whatever way he or she can participate. For example, one regular use of listening, speaking, reading, writing, and thinking is the making of a grocery list.

A very young child can be carried along while the adult is looking in the refrigerator and cupboards and deciding what needs to be purchased. Picking up an almost empty peanut butter jar, saying something like "Oh! I see we need more peanut butter," writing "peanut butter" on the grocery list, and then buying peanut butter at the grocery store upon consulting the list accomplishes a lot. First, the child has repeated chances to see the purposes for reading and writing. Second, the child hears "peanut butter," sees the words on the label, and has chances to make connections.

A slightly older child could be sent to the cupboard to see how much peanut butter there is and could be drawn into the decision about whether it is time to buy more. "How much peanut butter is here?" "Do you think you'll want a peanut butter sandwich for lunch tomorrow?" Being sent on an errand with a task to carry out heightens auditory memory processes; as the child can handle it, the number of items to remember can be increased. "Please go to the cupboard and see how much peanut butter and how much jelly we have" can be expanded into "Please go to the cupboard and check on the peanut butter, the jelly, the sugar, and the vanilla."

By the time the child reaches the middle and high school years, this could turn into "Please see what staples [probably a new word!] need to be replaced and write them on the list on the refrigerator."

The child does not need to know all the words the adult is using. In the process of learning language and adding to it, much inference-making is done, anyway. Most of us learn words in their contexts rather than from being given definitions for them. Many a hearing child has probably been confused by someone applying the word "staples" to necessities in the pantry, rather than to the metal pieces that hold paper together, but they figure it out. So can the child who is deaf or hard of hearing. It would be very hard to figure it out, though, without the background knowledge of basic ingredients that will grow over the years of participating in list-making and food-buying. The adult cannot just drop in new words at random, however, and schema theory's attention to overlapping and interlocking networks of words, ideas, and processes explains why. There needs to be some sense that the child is ready to make the new connection to the new word or words. Anyone who spends a good deal of time with the child will usually be in a good position to sense when the child is "ripe" for a new connection.

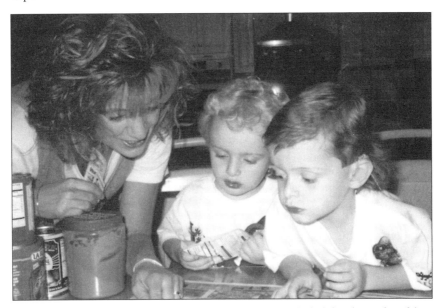

Figure 4.1. Everyone can participate! It's particularly helpful to have the object on hand while looking at the pictures and the writing and listening to the words for items on the list.

As the child begins to grasp the relationships between and among symbols, words, and objects, the adult might give the child a picture or a coupon for the item and ask her or him to locate it in the cupboard and, at an older age, in the grocery store. (Always be aware of supervision and safety concerns in both places. Children must be protected from falling off counters and from being carried off from grocery stores!) This gives the child real practice in matching objects and words. First, the picture of the peanut butter on a coupon matches some peanut butters, but not others, and so the child will learn that some discrimination is required. The patterns of the letters spelling out "peanut" and "butter" will become familiar over time, making this a good prereading activity.

Alerting Children to Symbols in the Environment

In the United States, one of the first written symbols children learn to identify is the symbol of a certain fast food restaurant (Ruddell & Ruddell, 1994, p. 91). Whatever we think of fast food restaurants, and whether we want to stop at them or not, we can make use of this phenomenon in promoting beginning reading. On a trip or in daily driving wherever the family lives, the child can be given the job of spotting symbols on signs that signify a promised stop somewhere. As development progresses, children can play the alphabet game, looking for the letters in alphabetical order on signs as they pass by — first, an "a" on a sign, then a "b" on another, and so on. Older children can be introduced to map reading and map-making and begin to take on some navigational responsibilities.

Bringing the child's attention to words and their printed forms is important. In order to surround the child with print, labels can be put on objects in the house. A card on the refrigerator can say "refrigerator" or "icebox" or "fridge" or whatever the family calls it. Tables, chairs, cabinets, the vacuum cleaner, and everything else can be labeled! That important discovery that "everything has a name" can be accompanied by the discovery that every name has a written representation. At the beginning, there is no need to dwell on how letters in the words sound or the ways the words look; many pre-readers begin to figure this out on their own as they construct for themselves how the system works.

Several sets of magnetic letters offer enough multiple letters to form many, many words and even simple sentences. Keeping them on the refrigerator makes them handy for play. Children and adults can move them around to make words, and adults can help with appropriate spellings when asked.

First Reading Words

An extension of the labeling of objects is the making of a collection of cards with the words the child requests from all the words he or she already knows in speaking, one word per card. Sylvia Ashton-Warner (1963) developed an approach to teaching Maori children in New Zealand which she called "organic teaching," meaning that what the children learned grew out of their own desire to learn. She developed her method when she found that European books did not fit the lives of her students. Not having Maori-oriented books, she turned to building her students' initial reading vocabularies (she called them "key vocabularies") by asking them which words they wanted to learn to read. In her words:

> *First words must have an intense meaning. First words must be already part of the dynamic life* (Ashton-Warner, 1963, p. 35).

Ashton-Warner's work stands out because her students were generally successful at reading in a society where most Maori did not find success in school. Her approach is applicable to the young child who is deaf or hard of hearing as well. The adult simply asks the child what words he or she wants to have written on cards and then makes a card for each word. Index cards work well for this. Together they go over the words with the adult telling the child what each one is as many times as is necessary. As the collection grows, the child begins to have some access to reading the words, resulting in control over the words he or she likes best. It might be tempting to turn this pile of cards into a pile of "flash cards" and then use them to "drill" the child, but this adult impulse should be resisted, unless the child takes the lead in doing so. Each word card can be treated as special, something to be read together, and something the child can take great pride in being able to identify. In working with the words, it will become apparent that various phonics cues, word shape cues, and experiential cues help the child remember what each word is. "See the 'm' at the beginning of the word? It says 'mm,' so the word is [the adult waits patiently] — mouse!" "Look at this word — it's [again, the patient wait] — house! See how it's like this one? [patient waiting] — mouse!" "Remember at Zach's house we saw a little animal in a cage? It was a — mouse!" Which cue to suggest will depend on the child's experience. Young children may remember that the card with the bent corner is the one that says "mouse." That is all right for the time being, though it's obviously not going to work as a permanent strategy for the school-age child. It is, however, a starting point, a symbol of one kind that stands for something else.

HOW DOES A CHILD KNOW WHAT A WORD IS?

It is important to keep in mind that young children generally do not know where one word begins and another ends. Conversation comes at us in streams of sounds, and breaking up the sounds into separate and regular parts, that is, into words, is part of the task of learning to read. This is part of what is being accomplished by labeling objects, pointing to words as we read aloud, and making word cards. But most important is remembering to have fun with the word cards. They can be shuffled and a few picked at random to make a funny story. They can be constructed in pairs and used for a concentration/memory game in which cards are laid face down and turned over one at a time. The task is to find the mate of each card by remembering what the cards look like because only two can be turned over at a time. When no match is made, the cards must be turned face down again, and the turn goes to the other player. Cards can also be paired with small objects or pictures that represent them. They can be put in alphabetical order. Sentences can be made from them. The child may choose to carry a favorite one around in a pocket. Punching a hole in each card and keeping them on a ring is a handy way to keep them together while also keeping it easy to take them off and put them back on as needed. For the older child, putting words to be remembered on cards to be pulled out for study can be a powerful study practice (Pauk, 1989, pp. 317-318).

Drawing the child into making a batch of cookies from a recipe or making anything that requires following written directions is another way of demon-

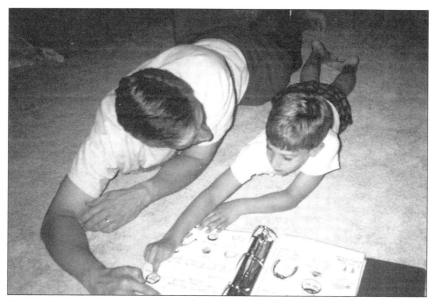

Figure 4.2. Reading the experience book together is an important daily literacy act.

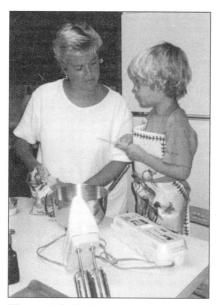 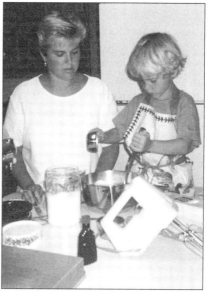

Figure 4.3. In these two pictures, the child is actively exploring the relationship between the words of the directions and the actions they represent.

strating that print is meaningful and important. The adult can read the directions aloud as the process unfolds. "Sift together $2^1/_4$ cups flour, 1 tsp. salt, and 1 tsp. baking soda" followed by helping the child fill the 1-cup measure twice and the $^1/_4$-cup measure once carries with it the powerful message that important information about where cookies come from is in the writing on the recipe card. Proceeding through the entire recipe together can bring the good feeling of accomplishment. As the ability to read grows, it can become the child's role to read the recipe aloud.

Table 4.1. Ways to Create a Rich Literacy Environment

1. Talk with, not at your child.

2. Attend to meaning before form.

3. Create real reasons for reading and writing: making and using lists; looking for highway signs; following written directions; writing a letter to grandparents.

4. Surround the child with print and bring it to the child's attention in ways that are fun for the child.

5. Attend to what the child wants to know about words.

6. Create and use language experience books.

7. Have many books and other reading material available.

8. Read to the child daily and make sure the child sees you reading for your own work and pleasure.

Using the Language Experience Book as a Beginning Reading Book

Ashton-Warner helped her students create what she called "transition readers" which were much like the language experience books I have discussed. These were books that were the children's own stories rather than the more culturally distant stories of others.

> First books must be made of the stuff of the child himself, whatever and wherever the child (Ashton-Warner, 1963, p. 35).

Language experience books, having been used to bring the child's attention to language, can be among the child's first reading books. Used as reading books, they make use of the language experience approach to reading. Descriptions of the language experience approach can be found in many books about the teaching of reading to young children. A source that I like is Durkin (1993) because of the flexibility she suggests in using the approach. Rather than giving prescriptive directions, Durkin suggests that the adult writer of each language experience story think about what the child seems ready for next in deciding how to use the child's words and what questions to ask the child in trying to extend the story. For example, if the child uses and seems ready to identify the names of various dinosaurs, then fit them in, even though each is a long and complex word. Essentially, in the language experience approach, much use is made of the child's language, so issues such as the teacher needing to decide whether the child is ready to learn to read this word or that word are not pertinent. Because the language comes mainly from the child, the child's choosing it demonstrates readiness to learn to read it.

In Chapter Three, I wrote that the purpose of the language experience book is to present natural language in a meaningful context and to stimulate exchanges of language in order to foster language acquisition and growth. In this chapter, I want to extend this to the child's learning to read. Learning to identify one's own words is much easier than learning to identify someone else's, because one's own words are already a part of oneself. The order of the words as well as the meaning they represent to the child are already a part of the child. Some memory for the words and their meaning is in place. A lot of the task is already complete! By using her or his own words, the child can make good use of an emerging understanding of what constitutes a word.

Ashton-Warner's insistence that "first books must be made of the stuff of the child himself" is supported by schema theory. The words the child dictates and the concepts they represent to the child come out of the network of stored understandings the child possesses at any given point, and so the reading of them taps into that same network. Any one of us as fluent readers must have sufficient background knowledge to bring to bear on anything we want to read and understand. This explains why, for example, most of us find reading and filling out an income tax form to be difficult. We do not do it with enough frequency to remember the steps from one time to the next, and most of us are not sufficiently familiar with how the language is being used in the directions to be able to figure out how to apply it to our own taxes. Yet, many of us have seen a professional tax return preparer sail through a form in a very short time! It is not because we are not good readers that we cannot understand the forms; it is that we have too little background knowledge to bring to bear on filling them out. Building the necessary background knowledge would enable us to cope with them. The content background knowledge needed by the child learning how to read must be very secure indeed, for he or she does not yet possess the procedural background knowledge of how reading works as a system. If nothing about the text taps into the knowledge the beginning reader possesses, then very little learning will go on. In order to learn something new, it must fit with something that is already known or what is already known must be changed in some way (Anderson, 1984, p. 255). The language experience approach depends on the premise that, when learning to read, it is easier to fit something in with what is already known than to change a previous understanding. Changing a previous understanding goes on all the time as the child learns about his or her environment and will be incorporated into the act of reading quite naturally as the process of reading becomes more secure; but such changes can get in the way of learning to read at the beginning, so it is best to start simply.

ESSENTIAL STEPS

The essential steps in using the language experience approach for reading instruction include:

1. Choose or allow the child to choose a significant event or subject to write about.
2. Draw a picture, have the child draw a picture, or use a photograph or picture obtained from another source (magazine, photocopy, etc.).
3. Ask the child to tell about it.
4. Write the child's words, usually in their exact form and order.
5. Read the words with the child.
6. Ask the child to read the words to you.
7. Return to the book frequently, just as you would to any beginning reading book.

Step 3 represents a transition in the use of the language experience book. When the child has learned enough language and can express her or himself in understandable ways, then the parent can ask for the child's own words at least part of the time, with the intent of working toward asking for the child's language most or all of the time. In general, the parent should write exactly the words the child offers. The question that always arises is whether the parent should write down the exact words if they are not "good" English. The answer to this depends on the developmental level of the child. For the child who is just beginning to put two words together to create a thought, it is sufficient to write the two words he or she offers. Writing "Baby crying" is fine for the young child who is just beginning to put two words together. For the child who has been doing so routinely, the adult might respond with "Oh, shall I write 'The baby is crying'?" Asking permission for what to write is a good way to check on the language level of the child, for the child who understands "The baby is crying" will accept the additional words; the child who doesn't may not. Remembering that it is difficult to identify words that do not make sense or which seem not to have a function helps in making this decision for this purpose. Asking to fill in a word or two in order to create a conventional sentence is fine, but rewording the entire sentence for the child is not. Taking the language experience book to the weekly or bi-weekly appointments with the language and speech therapist gives the therapist a chance to see something about where language therapy might proceed next, and so the parent may rest assured that the issue of learning standard language usage is being addressed.

As language experience books accumulate, they become good first reading books because they hold in rich and relevant ways the language of the child who will read them. These books become favorites because the main characters are the child and her or his family! The adult and the child can read them together just as they can read any other book together. Depending on the child's interest, the adult can point to the words as they are read by either the adult or the child, reinforcing the concept that words are separate entities. For this purpose, Durkin (1993, p. 112) suggests counting the words with the child to help develop this understanding. Gradually, the child will begin to identify the words by her or himself and can begin to read them with the help of the adult when a word or words cannot be remembered. For this purpose, it is usually best to just tell the child the unknown or forgotten word or words, rather than making a guessing game of it. Independence in reading the words will come with practice as more familiarity with them is established.

PRESSING ON

As time goes on, the adult can make more sophisticated suggestions about the words that will be written down. This would be in the same realm as the expansion of spoken language discussed in chapter four. Suppose the child offers, "Excited birthday!" on the day after her or his big birthday party. The parent could say, "Shall I write, 'I was very excited about my birthday party'?" Or if the child offers, "Exciting birthday," the parent might ask, "Do you want me to write, 'My birthday party was very exciting'?" Again, the words of the child should only be changed with the child's permission to do so. What if the child offers a sentence that breaks usage rules? "Tommy and me played on his slide at his house" could prompt the adult to say, "Most people would want to say 'Tommy and I.' Is that okay with you?"

Sometimes the adult will have to push the child a bit to get more than very short utterances to write in the language experience book. Asking questions such as, "What happened after you and Tommy played on the slide?" and "How did you and Tommy get so dirty?" could prompt more detailed sentences to record than ones with "yes" or "no" answers. Questions that ask how and why lead to sentences that represent more complex thought. While it is important to be able to relate a sequence of events ("We played on the swing after we played on the slide. Then we tried to catch the dog.") it is important to try to move toward more complex expression ("Dogs like to be petted, so we tried to catch Max. We fell in the mud. We'll be more careful next time we go after Max."). Asking questions to elicit more detail also helps expand the child's verbal expression. "Why does Max like to be petted? Where did the mud come from? What did it feel like? How high is the slide?"

The child who is deaf or hard of hearing will leave certain kinds of sounds and words out of his or her speech. These are usually sounds and words that are difficult to hear because they are of a frequency that the child does not hear well, or they are sounds and words not emphasized in conventional speaking by people with normal hearing. In the example above ("Baby crying") a young child may leave out "The" and "is" because he or she is at the two-word utterance stage, just as a child with normal hearing might do; he or she might leave these out at later stages because they are simply not heard and do not register. In this case, the adult will want to fill in the appropriate gaps, always asking if it is all right with the child to do so. ("People can understand you better if you say, 'The baby is crying.'") For many children, writing in the sounds and words that are not heard is the first signal that they are even present in people's speaking. At this point, reading and writing can begin to inform, and improve, listening and speaking.

Working Toward Language Learning Is Your Primary Task

In my studies of the reading and writing achievement of children who learned language and speech through the auditory-verbal approach, I learned that all but one child had been read to daily by a parent, and that all the parents had worked very hard to create a language-enriched environment. The task of the parent of the preschooler, then, is to work hard toward language learning and to present as much meaningful spoken and written language as possible to the child so as to prepare her or him for formal instruction in reading at school. As I have said, it is not necessary to send the child to school already knowing how to read — though that would be a plus — but sending the child with good language ability, knowledge of how books are constructed, and the ability to identify some letters and words will provide the teacher the necessary foundation with which to work with the child. Without being prompted, the great majority of parents whom I have interviewed observed that their child had good ability to focus on the task at hand and was able to spend considerable time paying attention during any instructional period. These abilities are prized in their students by kindergarten and first grade teachers, and they seem to be an important by-product of auditory-verbal therapy and the one-on-one attention the child gets through listening, speaking, reading, and writing with an adult. Children learn to read by reading, through having repeated and meaningful contact with reading materials for which they have sufficient background knowledge. It is not necessary to drill them in letter names or phonics rules for "sounding out" words. The best approach for the parent of a beginning reader is to read with the child every day.

Picture Books to Chapter Books — and Beyond!

A natural progression of reading begins with the reading of pictures in the language experience book and the reading of manufactured picture books. The child who is in an environment where there is easy access to and encouragement to explore many interesting materials will work up from the easy through the harder materials, usually without much prompting. Staying with one sort of reading for a while probably signals that the child feels there is more to be learned from it (Lewis & Long, 1991). As long as there are more challenging and interesting materials available, and adults and older children demonstrate that they value them, most children will seek them out as they are ready to do so.

A Note on Later Language and Reading Development

A finding of my second study is that Gates-MacGinitie Reading Test scores showed the middle school students who are deaf or hard of hearing to be reading less well than their hearing peers, while most of the elementary and high school students' scores were above average in comparison with their hearing peers (Robertson, under review). Of course, it is possible that the middle school students I tested were lower achievers when they were in their elementary years and that they will be lower achievers in high school. It is possible that the elementary and high school students in my study have been and will always be higher achievers. I do not know, for in this study I did not follow the same students throughout their schooling.

I do, however, think something else of great interest is operating with these students. My current interpretation is that the middle school tests draw from a far wider set of words than do earlier tests, which causes the student who is deaf or hard of hearing not to perform as well on them because their vocabularies are still limited in certain ways compared with students with normal hearing. This is important because as one looks toward the future of a child who is deaf or hard of hearing, it can be helpful to know there will be predictable ups and downs in achievement as measured by standardized tests. Further study is needed, but for now I think my interpretation is helpful in planning for an individual student's education.

Interestingly, almost half the middle school students experienced a significant gap between their comprehension scores and their vocabulary scores. By this I mean that the middle school students I tested had scores that were significantly higher for the comprehension portion of the Gates-MacGinitie Reading Test than for the vocabulary portion. Both elementary and high school students I tested had comprehension and vocabulary scores that were more balanced in relation to each other. In comparison to middle school students with normal hearing, these children who are deaf or hard of hearing appeared to have more limitations on their vocabularies than on their comprehension.

I interpret these results with some caution as demonstrating that learning language is a long-term project. The middle school students showed themselves to be relatively good at comprehension in the presence of lesser vocabularies. They were able to make some sense of what they were given to read even when they did not know all the words. The middle school student with normal hearing has had far more access to words in the environment than has the student who is deaf or hard of hearing and so has a larger working vocabulary to bring to the task of a reading test. The student who is deaf or hard of hearing at this age is simply behind compared to the student with normal hearing in learning the large variety of words that could show up on a standardized reading test. The student has to use all his or her powers of guessing based on fewer language clues in order to answer the questions.

The good news is that, by the time the students get to high school, it is predictable that they will have caught up in their vocabulary-building, and this will, in turn, help them catch up on comprehension tasks. This catching up probably happens as the student continues to use reading to learn new words and ideas and continues to improve in her or his ability to talk with others. It is important that seeing lower standardized test scores does not cause parents, therapists, and teachers to begin to expect less of the child who is deaf or hard of hearing. If progress is taking place for the child, then pressing on with the approach should produce good results, even though they may take longer to appear. Just as we had to wait for those first spoken words and sentences, we have to wait for development of reading vocabulary even as we do all we can to nurture it.

5
Can My Child Learn To Write Well?

Highlights

▼ Children who are deaf or hard of hearing can become good writers.

▼ Good achievement in listening and reading usually leads to good achievement in writing.

▼ In the presence of many examples of writing, children construct an understanding of how the writing system works.

▼ The language experience book can become a beginning writing book.

▼ Children learn to write by using writing for real purposes.

Studying the Writing Achievement of Auditory-Verbal Learners

PEOPLE WHO DO NOT READ WELL ALSO DO NOT WRITE WELL, PEOPLE WHO ARE DEAF or hard of hearing included. Given that most people with prelingual deafness read at much lower levels than people with normal hearing, expectations of writing ability are lower for the person who is deaf or hard of hearing.

Reasoning that one's reading achievement predicts one's writing achievement to some extent, I included writing achievement of children who had learned language through the auditory-verbal approach as an additional focus of my second study. As I described in chapter one, I asked each child in fourth grade and older to produce a short writing sample after completing the Gates-MacGinitie reading test. Each student was given the simple direction to "write about something that interests you" and had the opportunity to talk with me about the choice of topic if he or she wanted to do so. Most responded with "Is it all right if I write about _____?" to which I responded, "Sure. Fine." Their topics ranged from "My Best Friend" to "The Roller Coaster" to science fiction.

In the normal school setting, especially at the elementary level, testing of children is ordinarily carried out over a period of days or even weeks, with different parts of a test being given at different times. Since I was able to meet with each child or adolescent only one time, I had to ask for an unusual sustaining of focus and energy from each of them directly after the reading test. In addition, tests of writing that are in greatest use currently provide time and directions for the test-taker to write a draft and to revise it before handing it in to be scored. There was not time for the students I tested to do this, and so their writing samples were first drafts. For both of these reasons I was concerned that their writing achievement might not look adequate because it would be judged on the basis of incomplete work. In short, adequate or proficient writers might not be able to demonstrate their abilities given the testing situation.

In the education world, official evaluations of student writing are done usually by teachers highly experienced with this task. Writing samples are collected and sent to groups of teachers who have had a great deal of experience in deciding which papers rank high and which rank low. It is done this way because the evaluation of writing involves so many variables that can be described in generalities but that cannot be pinned down with absolute precision. The evaluation of writing cannot be standardized in the same way that responses to questions about reading a particular passage can be; that is, there are no exact words or phrases that can be expected of all good writers responding to the same prompt. Neither can all good writers be expected to produce a specifiable number of sentences or even to use a prescribed format for sentences or the work as a whole. A current approach to the evaluation of writing begins with an agreed-upon holistic scale which is developed through conversation about what is valued in students' writing at various levels. Then evaluators read the papers in relation to the holistic scale, choosing papers that fit the criteria of each position on the scale as representatives of those positions. Despite the fact that there is a certain amount of subjectivity involved in reading the writing of another, the evaluation of writing according to established criteria is in widespread use (for example, in state proficiency tests, the Scholastic Achievement Test and certain Advanced Placement tests). I made use of such an approach in trying to determine how well the students were writing compared to students with normal hearing at the time they were tested and turned to teachers in the county where I live who do such evaluation routinely.

I had each writing sample typed exactly the way it was written so that handwriting was not an issue in the judging of the samples. Misspellings, misuses of words, and unconventional word orders were not corrected, though Canadian spellings were changed to U.S. spellings and geographical cues were deleted so that the readers would not be influenced by them.

Then I mixed the samples I had gathered with "anchor papers" from a county-level coalition of school districts where teachers and administrators have worked for many years to evaluate and improve their students' writing. The "anchor papers" are papers they have collected over time from each grade level that represent four scores, or achievement levels of writing, as determined by a large number of evaluators in numerous evaluations over many years. These teachers refer to their evaluation process as "holistic grading" because they look at each paper as a whole in relation to agreed-upon criteria in order not to get bogged down in small details about the writing. They are interested mainly in determining an overall score for each paper that represents how well it communicates with its reader.

For each grade level for which I had samples, the samples were put into a pile along with two Level 1 papers, two Level 2 papers, two Level 3 papers, and two Level 4 papers, none of which carried a mark or a score. Not wanting to give any of the teacher/evaluators any reason to prejudge what they were to read, I did not tell them they would be reading the writing of students who are deaf or hard of hearing or that they would be reading "anchor papers," though I thought some might recognize them; I just asked two experienced teachers from each grade level to read, score, and respond to the papers as part of a study I was doing. For all they knew, I could have been studying their reading of the papers!

I was interested first in whether the teachers would give the "anchor papers" the scores they had been given originally. If that measure stayed steady, then I felt I could have some confidence in the teachers' ratings of the papers of the students who are deaf or hard of hearing. Upon finding no statistically significant difference in their ratings of the anchor papers, I moved on.

HOW WELL DID THE AUDITORY-VERBAL STUDENTS WRITE?

Only three writing samples collected from the 23 students who are deaf or hard of hearing in grades 4 through 14 (grades 13 and 14 represent the first two years of college) were judged to be unacceptable (scored as "1") for their grade level; one of them was written by an elementary student, and two were by high school students. The scores ranged from "4" (highest) to "1" (lowest) and were distributed as follows: Of two 4th–5th graders, one scored a "3" and the other scored a "1." Of nine 6th–8th graders, three scored "3" and six scored "2." Of 12 9th–14th graders, three scored "4," three scored "3," four scored "2," and two scored "1." These numbers can be seen in Table 5.1, as well.

Levels 2, 3, and 4 represent varying degrees of acceptability, with Level 4 representing the highest achievement for the grade level. A Level 4 paper shows careful

Table 5.1. Writing Scores for 23 Students, Grades 4 through 14*

Score	4-5	6-8	9-14	
4			3	
3	1	3	3	
2		6	4	Passing
1	1		2	

Grade Level

* The first two years of college are included as Grades 13 and 14.

organization; good and varied vocabulary; a sense of purpose and under-standing of what is necessary to say to be understood (this can be described as a sense of audience); good sentence structure; few errors in mechanics, usage, grammar, and spelling; and creativity and originality. Levels 3 and 2 show lesser, but not unacceptable achievement in all those areas, and level 1 rates the sample poor in all the areas. The actual holistic rating scale can be found in Appendix I. In the group of students I tested, there is a clear trend toward increasing mastery of written language as years in school increase, as can be seen in the higher proportion of "4's" and "3's" scored by the high school students.

WHAT DID THE TEACHERS NOTICE ABOUT THE AUDITORY-VERBAL STUDENTS' WRITING?

I was also interested in knowing more specifically what the teachers thought about the language used in the samples, and so I asked them to fill out the fol-lowing checklist for each sample:

Does this paper have:

_____1. Phrasings and/or tone characteristic of the conversational style of the writer's age group.

_____2. Phrasings and/or tone characteristic of the writing style often used in books read by the writer's age group.

_____3. Phrasings and/or tone characteristic of the writing style often used in school books read by the writer's age group.

_____4. Use of language or punctuation that indicates the writer is begin-ning to use more sophisticated language but that he or she hasn't quite mastered it yet.

_____5. Use of language or punctuation that indicates the writer is not a mainstream user of English.

More middle school students were noted as using conversational style in their writing, possibly indicating something of a surge in their listening abilities. It was clear they were writing the language they were hearing in their environ-ment. Given the social-developmental tasks that preadolescent and young ado-lescent children need to master, the character of their writing makes the lan-guage use in these samples look very normal in comparison to their peers with normal hearing. Some examples of their conversational writing include: "He is really cute!"; "I am totally crazy about animals"; and "Well, that's allllll about me!" High school papers were also noted as containing conversational style, though this style does not stand out as prominently among the qualities the teachers noted about those papers as it does for the middle school papers.

I have noticed in my conversations over the years with children and adults who are deaf or hard of hearing who were proficient readers that at least some of their word choices and phrasings sounded as though they came from the books they read, and so I wanted to see whether that would show up in their writing. The teachers found both general book language and schoolbook lan-guage in the writing samples across the grades, from grade 5 through grade 14.

Examples of book language in the students' writing include: "I like them because they are interesting." (from a 5th grader) and "Before I go any further, let me . . ." (from a 6th grader). Comments on samples from grades 11, 12, and 13 concerning schoolbook language included "very sophisticated for 11th grade — in terms of style, organization"; "very formal tone"; "the vocabulary is sophisticated" in describing such sentences as "On the other hand, there are those who deserve the title of professor/teacher, etc. These teachers are open to new ideas and methods of fostering maximum student/teacher interaction." This quality in the students' writing is important because it demonstrates the power of reading in shaping the language a person uses, both in writing and in speaking. For the person who is deaf or hard of hearing who may be missing a certain amount of what is spoken around her or him, being able to use reading as a source of language and information is a way to fill in the gaps created by the hearing loss. A beneficial cycle of literacy is set up: listening prepares for reading and writing which in turn prepare for listening, and so on.

Growing sophistication in language use was noted by the teacher/evaluators beginning with the 6th grade samples and extending through grade 14. This was explained to the teacher/evaluators as language that was just beyond an age group's usual usage, or use of language that is not "quite right," but that suggests the writer is on the verge of being able to use it appropriately. Such growth at all levels indicates a continuing interest in words and how to use them on the part of the students; it also points to their genuine desire to increase their own abilities and their willingness to take risks in how they express themselves. Teacher/evaluators noticed such sentences as these: "Another trail called Parsenn Bowl, is, too located in Winter Park and is new to the area, because it is challenging"; and "Graduation leads on to better things in life and therefore going onwards with your life." Both these sentences are awkward, yet they communicate a great deal and signal a desire toward complex expression. They may also be first draft sentences which would have been improved had the students had time to revise their writing. Teacher/evaluators expressed admiration of the older students' growing ability to use colons and semicolons, complex sentence structure, and words such as "sentient," "discontented," "manifested," and "pondered."

People who have difficulty with language speak and write in ways that show they are having trouble, and their expression often looks as though it comes from a person who has come from another culture, who perhaps knows another language and is just now struggling with English. Imagine transplanting yourself to France having had a year or so of French in high school. It would be very hard to sound well educated! This is often the plight of the person who is deaf or hard of hearing because he or she must at times operate with an incomplete understanding of the language of the environment. Examples of language that appeared to have been written by a student whose main language might not be English included: "he love to ride" and "he ride" (grade 5); "In the park, they were so crowded in this park because the weathers hasn't been warming enough in these seasons" (grade 6); and "she say that next week it will be the test Tuesday" (grade 7). All of these sentences show irregularities in grammatical structure that signal a lack of knowledge of English. The inability to hear the sound of "s" consistently is reflected in each sentence, as well. Beyond grade 8, the samples were free of such irregularities, suggesting that by about that time the students had gained good facility with the structure of English.

Not one teacher/evaluator suspected the samples as coming from some special group of students who would usually be thought incapable of normal achievement. The students' writing did not look different overall to the teacher/evaluators compared to the writing of students with normal hearing at each grade level with whom they usually deal, attesting to the very normal development of language in this group of children and adolescents who are deaf or hard of hearing.

Writing Development Parallels Reading Development

Just as reading is not simply the converting of written symbols to sounds, writing is not just the translation of sounds to symbols. Once we understand that reading grows out of listening and speaking, it becomes apparent that writing develops in concert with reading. Using this orientation, then, it can be said that the task for young children learning to write is that of figuring out their language's conventional system of letters and their patterns in order to represent what they want to convey (Ferreiro, 1991, pp. 31-56).

Beginning writing can be said to be taking place with the first scribbles on paper, the wall, or, alas, your favorite book. This scribbling is entirely necessary and represents a time of practice and hypothesis testing on the part of the child about how the system of writing works. We want children to scribble or write in appropriate places, of course, and so we need to be alert to their needs to express themselves. Providing paper and crayons and supervision for using them goes a long way in supporting the need of the child for expression — and in keeping our walls relatively free of experimentation! Learning how to write one's own name and the names of important people in one's life often serves as a first step to literacy. As Ashton-Warner's (1963, 1986) experience demonstrates, such personal words hold extraordinary power. For many children personal words are so fascinating that they provide the fundamental insight that some kind of relationship exists between the shape of the letters and the saying of the word. In our home we have preserved two such examples of Annie's experiments. With great delight, I remember her being enormously excited about writing her name. I watched the process with real interest as Annie tried out different ways of representing the "A" and the "i," especially. For a while she wrote her name on everything she could, and I thought we had been successful at making sure it was all done in acceptable places. Sometime later I found that she had written her name inside my bedroom closet and on the wall in the laundry room. Rather than becoming angry, I felt — and still feel, because I haven't allowed them to be painted over — a real sense of fondness and wonder. We are lucky to have remained in the same house where we still have a charming record of her emerging literacy.

Responding to Your Child's Writing (Even if it Looks Like Scribbling to You)

When a child takes scribbles or a picture he or she has drawn to an adult, the kind of response the adult makes can enhance or detract from the child's developing sense of what it means to make marks on paper. If the adult says, "Tell me about what you have drawn (or written) here," it is a signal for the child to "read" the symbols for the adult. Never mind that the child may explain the same scribblings in different ways to different people. At this point the child is working on the concept that the scribblings can stand for something that is real somewhere else. He or she is learning that marks on paper can convey meanings and is experimenting with various possibilities.

Spending time daily with books, stories, and words — in short, with anything in print or handwriting — provides models for writing that the child can do. There is much to be learned about all the different ways letters and sounds can be represented, about where one word stops and another begins, about punctuation and capitalization, about what kinds of words follow other kinds of words, and about how stories and descriptions of processes, places, and things proceed. At the beginning, a child can learn much by being in the presence of well-formed language found in interesting materials and pictures. The adult will do well to trust that the child is paying attention to the attributes that answer some question concerning language that is compelling and necessary to her or him at each contact with written language (Lewis & Long, 1991). Later, in school, formal instruction can set forth the rules for carrying out conventional modes of expression. It is easier for the child to learn the conventional rules if he or she has first experienced the language in meaningful ways so that there are schematic frameworks in which to put the rules. Instruction that begins with the rules will be harder to comprehend.

Using the Language Experience Book to Help Your Child Write

James Britton points out that we use language not only to communicate with others but also to make sense of our own experiences and that once the child begins going away from home to school, for even part of a day, he or she has a real need to use language for both of these reasons (Britton, 1993, p. 71). At this point the language experience book can take on an additional function, that of being a place where the adult can write down the words of the child about something that occurred when the child was away from the adult during school, an outing, or playtime at another child's house. For perhaps the first time, the adult will not know what the child has done during a period of time, and so there is real need for communication to take place. From the child's point of view, there is a parallel authentic need to put words together to describe to the adult what has happened in the time apart. The language experience book can be used as the place where the adult records the words of the child about those experiences. One advantage the adult can have that the child will not have to know about is that the adult can have a conversation with the teacher or the caregiver or the parent of the playmate and so can know about significant events of the day in order to understand what the child is trying to convey. It is helpful to keep a notebook in which teachers and others can write to the parent about such things so that the parent has a context for the child's words which may be very difficult to understand as the child is acquiring language and speech. We did this often with Annie and avoided a lot of frustration on her part because we could almost always piece together what she was saying because we knew something about her experiences apart from us. Recall the research by Schlesinger (1988) in which she demonstrates how important the responses of the adult are to the child. Whenever the adult can understand the child's utterances and take them seriously enough to write them down, confidence is built in the child as a comprehender and as a communicator.

Before the child can do the writing for her or himself, the adult does the actual production of words on the pages, but it is the child who is producing the words, and so it is the child who is the writer. As the child begins to learn how to produce the words on paper, he or she can gradually take over the role of scribe. There may be a time when the child "writes" or draws in the book and the adult prints neatly next to the "writing" or drawing the words that the child says. The adult can see her or himself as the nurturing facilitator, helping a lot at the beginning and all the while working toward independence in writing for the child.

As I wrote in Chapter Four, the question of whether the adult should correct misused words in the child's writing has many answers. In general when the child is holding the pencil and doing the actual writing, if it is close in character to conventional writing and is not just scribbling where the adult might "translate" in conventional writing below the scribbles, the adult should let the child have control over the production of the text. Too much interference by the adult can cause the child to label her or himself as incapable of learning this process and result in a giving up which will then provide proof of being incapable. However much one wants to reach out and make the words look right, the temptation should be resisted. Remembering that the language experience book is part of a long-term process and that at this point the child is at the beginning of that process is helpful in resisting that temptation. There is no need for the language experience book to be a flawlessly written record of the child's experiences. It is a learning tool, one whose pages will be cherished in later years for their unique qualities.

The entries in the book written by the child must also be among the reading texts for the child. Reading one's own writing is important. First, it is easy to read because it is familiar and predictable. Second, reading the child's writing with her or him provides the child control and pride in the process which inspire self-confidence. Third, reading one's own writing leads eventually to revising one's own writing, a habit which should be cultivated for it will be extremely valuable to the student in later years, for it leads to better thinking.

Writing for Real Communication Needs

As the child spends time with the adult who is writing frequently in the child's presence in order to complete meaningful tasks, the child will begin to emulate this behavior. Yetta Goodman (1990, p. 118) reminds us that children learn best through playing and that playing at learning to write is no exception. Playing at being grown-up helps children conceptualize their world and make sense of it. While we may usually think about this in terms of copying the actions of the mail carrier, the farmer, or the parent in play situations, copying adults using reading and writing is an important step.

My husband Mike happened onto a good example of this when he started playing what he and Annie called "Taco Bell." They would stack up cardboard bricks to simulate the counter at Taco Bell and then take turns being the customer and being the person behind the counter. The customer would say what he or she wanted and the counter person would "write" it down with a pretend pencil on pretend paper and then go and get the pretend order. Sometimes they would wear hats and aprons, sometimes not. The value of the game was in giving Annie the steps to follow (the schema) in going to a restaurant with a counter where she would have to speak intelligibly and meaningfully in order to get what she wanted. She got to try both roles in the schema and could see that writing down the order (even though that is not how fast food places operate actually) is useful.

As she grew older, she and her friends would sometimes treat us to snacks and then later to dinners they would make, where the first step would be the writing of a menu, followed by the taking of our order which they wrote down and followed. Playing at these grownup roles has given them great satisfaction and self confidence. Noticing how people in the child's life use writing for real purposes can lead to the creation of many games such as our "Taco Bell" game. Parents make lists and write letters, waiters take orders, clerks in stores write down information, reporters take notes for a story, new friends write down each other's address and telephone number, people take messages for each other, doctors write prescriptions, and so on. Pretending to do these actions and switching roles in the game establishes each of these communicative procedures as a schema in the child's memory network of social interactions and plays up the purpose of writing within them.

The parent can help the child write letters, lists, notes, titles — anything that needs to be written, first by enlisting the child's attention when the adult is doing such a task for a real purpose, and later by aiding the child in doing the task for her or his own purpose. "I'm writing a letter to Grandma and Grandpa. What shall I write for you?" might be a way to start. "Shall I tell them about your ride on the horse?" "Okay, what shall I say?" "Let's draw a picture to go with it."

Later this could become, "Let me help you write a letter to Grandma and Grandpa," as the adult transfers the task of writing to the child who is developing the ability to put letters and words on paper.

An occasion such as a birthday or a holiday provides many opportunities for writing. "Who shall we invite to your birthday party? How about making a list? . . . What shall we have to eat? . . . We need to write it down. . . . Let's make some invitations. . . . Here's where we put the address on the envelope. . . . Let's go mail the invitations. . . . Here's a message that Jamie can come to your party. . . . Grandma and Grandpa want some ideas for a present that you would like. . . . Let's make a wish list for them. . . . It's time to write some thank-you notes for all your presents."

Getting ready to go on a trip can require listing clothes to take, writing notes to the neighbors to look after the mail, and listing places to visit. When a batch of pictures comes back from being developed, the adult can draw the child into writing labels for them in the photo album. The child can help organize toys and help decide labels for shelves where different kinds of toys will be kept.

In almost every endeavor there is an opportunity to write for meaningful purposes. Parents often simply take care of such matters themselves so as to minimize the confusion that any occasion can produce. Children who are deaf or hard of hearing (and those with normal hearing) can benefit greatly from being drawn into such planning and learning how to use writing to produce a result of some kind.

Reading as a Springboard for Writing

Keep in mind that all the list-making, note-taking, letter writing, story writing, and labeling should be going on in an environment where the reading of the lists, notes, letters, stories, and labels is taking place along with the regular reading of storybooks. Many children, deaf or hard of hearing or not, construct for themselves a usable rationale for how the letters and words are related based on their emerging knowledge of language patterns that include word order, sounds, and shapes of letters and words (Durkin, 1966). These patterns become dependable in their memories and lead to the building of more memories of patterns. The adult in the situation must think carefully about and be alert to relationships between reading and writing and be ever ready to make ordinary events into chances for the child to learn about them. The child who has been in a word-rich environment should be very ready for (and may not even need) the formal reading instruction offered in the early grades.

6

What Can Parents, Therapists, and Teachers Do at Various Levels of Schooling?

Highlights

▼ The goal of those working with young children who are deaf or hard of hearing is to get them ready for school.

▼ Parents, therapists, and teachers should take a team approach in helping children who are deaf or hard of hearing.

▼ Knowing the individual child's knowledge and modes of expression is important in nurturing further development.

▼ Children with and without deafness learn at different paces.

▼ Children use their background knowledge to interpret what they read and express themselves when they write.

▼ All language work must be meaningful.

The Goal of Preparing the Child for Learning

THE PARENT OF THE CHILD WHO IS DEAF OR HARD OF HEARING SHOULD AIM TO DO exactly what the parent of any other child should aim to do regarding the child's education. He or she should do everything possible to help the child arrive at first grade healthy, happy, and with good self-esteem. The child should have acquired as much spoken language as possible by having used hearing aids or a cochlear implant. Learning to use whatever hearing the child has results in the growth and development of the auditory brain centers that such technologies access. The child who wants to learn and who arrives at school ready to do so will learn readily, regardless of where he or she is in developmental terms upon beginning. All of the therapy and activities in a confidence-building, nurturing environment during the preschool years combine to produce readiness to learn.

It is not unusual for children who are deaf or hard of hearing and who learn language and speech through the auditory-verbal approach to arrive in school still not able to put many words together in speech. I learned this in talking with the parents of the children I tested and can report that this was Annie's experience as well. It must be taken into consideration that a lag in language development is normal for these children. After all, most were quite likely deprived of hearing all language until they received hearing aids or a cochlear implant and then needed time to listen to language in the environment before beginning to speak, just as a child with normal hearing must do. Therefore, a 3-year-old child aided or implanted at age two may be two years or more behind in language development (Flexer, 1994, p. 15). It is unlikely that this deficit can be made up entirely in time for school, but that is not a reason not to try. Much can and should be accomplished before the child begins school. Children learn a great deal from each other because the motivation to understand and be understood by one's classmates is quite powerful. Putting the child who is deaf or hard of hearing in daily contact with children with normal hearing can contribute much to bringing a child's language development along. It is well known that "children learn in social settings and not in isolation" (Ferreiro, 1990, p. 24).

Therefore, the parent of a child who is deaf or hard of hearing should look for a school setting which continues the language enriched-environment that has been created at home, in speech and language therapy, and, if applicable, in preschool. In Ferreiro's (1990) words, this is the best "literacy environment" for the child. Such a school environment will offer continuous opportunity to learn language by listening to it and reading it and by using it in speaking and writing. Each child will be surrounded with speech and with print and will have ample materials and opportunities available for writing. Children will be encouraged to speak and listen to each other, not just to the teacher.

Thinking in Terms of a Team

The questions of what type of school, what kind of first grade, and placement with which teacher are always going to be matters of individual need and preference. The parent can make the best decisions by becoming as informed as possible concerning all the options available and by thinking of himself or her-

self as part of the team that will work together throughout the formal education of the child. While it may be tempting after all the work of therapy and
working with the child seemingly every waking hour in the preschool years, the
parent should not think her or his work is done when the process of formal
education begins. The parent cannot rest, yet, and leave it all to the school.
This is the time for the parent to become a monitor of what is happening with
the child, while continuing to do the language and speech building he or she
has been doing.

It is a good idea for the parent to get to know school personnel as early as
possible so that the team can form on behalf of the child. It is good for the
school to know several years in advance, if possible, that the child will be attending there. That way the decision-makers will have time to get used to the idea,
and they will be less fearful of taking on what may feel to them to be a new challenge. The team need not be gathered together formally or even designated
formally as a team, though much can be gained if that is done. The child may
or may not qualify as needing a formal Individual Education Plan (IEP), but if
he or she does, then the parents should welcome this process and become an
integral part of it. A broader team should include the teacher(s), the principal,
the school psychologist, the speech and language teacher, the school secretary,
an itinerant teacher of the deaf or hard of hearing, the audiologist, the therapist, and the parent(s). As the child grows older, he or she becomes part of the
team, participating as fully as possible at each developmental level in her or his
education. All members of the team need to communicate clearly and frequently with each other so that all understand the child's changing needs.
Notes written in a notebook that circulates among the members of the team
provide information to everyone and contribute to documenting the child's
progress. Informal conversations and formal team meetings are also necessary.
Just as the parent of the young child who is deaf or hard of hearing is often
able to understand the child's speaking when others cannot (because he or she
knows the content of most of the child's experiences), so can the team members come to know about the child's experiences in order to understand the
child's speaking. As the years go by, the composition of the team will change
depending on the child's needs, but the parent should always see her or himself as part of an educational team rather than as sole director of the child's
education or as a person who cannot contribute anything to the process. Good
communication among team members is crucial, because if trust breaks down
and an adversarial relationship develops, the child's possibilities shrink.

Working with the Child's Developmental Level and Knowledge Base

In working with any learner, regardless of the learner's age and ability to hear,
the teacher needs to be aware of each individual's developmental level and
knowledge base. "The teaching procedures for each level consist of being
aware of what characterizes the thoughts of a child at a particular point in

time" (Grossi, 1990, p. 112). Such awareness enables the teacher to understand an off-beat answer and to see kernels of understanding where full understanding is not yet present. In such instances the teacher can then provide explanations which build the necessary background knowledge for more complete understanding. The teacher must learn to keep in mind that the child who is deaf or hard of hearing may have missed out on hearing crucial information that can be taken for granted in children with normal hearing. Once that information is understood by the child who is deaf or hard of hearing, progress can be made. If that piece remains lacking, progress will be impeded. Another way of thinking about this is to turn to Vygotsky's concept of a zone of proximal development (Vygotsky, 1962, p. 103; Britton, p. 305).

Vygotsky's theory is that learning takes place through a continuous process of adding on the next bit of information. Such information can be about how to do something or it can be information containing content. The ground must be laid for information new to the learner to be added, and when that is done, new ground is available for the next bit of information. The zone of proximal development is that area in which the learner is now ready to learn with some help, and it represents the next and best place for the learner to add information. Vygotsky's theorizing centers on learning as a social activity, and so adding information is seen as a social process in which the learner interacts with another person who could be an adult or a child. An alert adult can facilitate learning by being aware of what the child knows so that he or she can help the child fit the next part in with what is already known. In the words of Hansen and Graves (1992), "Thus it is up to the adult to find out what the child needs and/or wants. This information is what is most learnable."

Keeping in mind that people have zones of proximal development in all areas of knowing, an example of it in reading would be the discovery of compound words. The child who knows "can" and "not" might be confused upon encountering "cannot," but the groundwork is laid for reading and understanding it. The adult can help the child discover how "can" and "not" fit together to form "cannot" both in representation in letters and in meaning. Next for an individual child might be the discovery of contractions: "cannot" can also be expressed as "can't." The progression of this learning is not set in stone, yet it is not random either, as each child makes progress that is logical for her or him individually. Every child has different experiences and so has different information about processes and content stored in memory. Some children will be ready for and will absorb "can't" before learning "cannot," for example.

Making sure that learning keeps happening appears to be a formidable task, a task similar to the programming of a computer, and it would be, if the adult had to think about every single bit of information that needed to be "fed into" the child. Luckily, individual human beings are usually able to select the next logical bit of information and fit it with what is already known, taking in the information that answers questions he or she has while being in contact with a given experience or material. Quite likely you have had the experience of an "aha moment," that instant when you realized some new connection.

Children probably have "aha moments" all the time if their environment is stimulating, because so much is new to them, and they have so much connection-making to do. Yet, children are not confused by having to learn so much. They are continuously building and refining theories in their heads with which to make sense of the world around them (Smith, 1978, pp. 57-58). The best way to help this process along is to create an environment which is rich in meaning. This is the reason for the conventional wisdom of the "literacy environment," for having many books, interesting toys, and craft supplies available to the child. It is the reason for the advice that the adult participate in the exploration of such materials with the child. It also accounts for why children do not always learn what we think they should have learned from a particular lesson or experience; they may have been busy taking in something else that was in their zone of proximal development at the time.

Language Learning is Functional and Social, Variable, and Coherent

The task during the school years from preschool through high school is one of helping the child who is deaf or hard of hearing to continue the process of catching up in language development in relation to her or his peers with normal hearing. Some gaps may remain throughout this time, particularly gaps in vocabulary. As the students I have tested demonstrate, however, some who are deaf or hard of hearing can even surpass the reading and writing achievement of students with normal hearing. The implications for what must happen in the school setting are many; in general, an essential quality of a beneficial school curriculum is that it be based on many kinds of communication between and among teachers, students, and materials. Naomi Baron's (1995) observations that language learning is functional and social (p. 130); variable (p. 131); and coherent (p. 131) are helpful in developing criteria for what should be happening throughout the school years.

LANGUAGE LEARNING IS FUNCTIONAL AND SOCIAL

A school curriculum that is functional and social helps students get along in their own overlapping worlds. It satisfies each student's needs and helps her or him relate what can be learned abstractly to what is present in her or his life. Material is chosen for its relevance and applicability to real-life activities. For example, at the elementary level this could be carried out in a study of the roles of various people in the community. What does the mail carrier do? How about the firefighter? The mayor? Middle school students could interview people in their families in order to find out about personal memories of particular historical periods in the United States and other countries. High school students could discover and research a problem in the community, determine how to act on it, and use writing to their government representatives and writing to the local newspaper in seeking a solution. In carrying out any of these areas of study, the students will have to use conversation in conjunction with the reading of sources beyond themselves. Such learning is functional because it connects students to information that matters to them in their own lives; it is social because the work involves communicating with others. These aspects are important in fostering increasingly more complex use of language in all its forms. It is much easier to learn words which are applicable to one's own life and interests and which enable one to communicate with people with whom one is usually in contact.

LANGUAGE LEARNING IS VARIABLE

A school curriculum which recognizes that language learning is variable for different children and for the individual child at different times is less likely to insist that all children learn the same material at the same time. Earlier theories that suggested that all children go through the same essential stages have been amended as researchers have discovered pronounced rate and style differences among children (Baron, p. 131). This discovery benefits the child who is deaf or hard of hearing especially because teachers no longer need to require that all the children in a classroom be working in the same way on the same page of the same material. Once it is recognized that every learner in the classroom is by definition at a different place in her or his development, there is room in that classroom for the child who is deaf or hard of hearing whose language abilities are unevenly developed, just as there is room in that classroom for any other child, because all the children will be at different places in their development. Social interaction among peers with differing language skills fosters language development in all the children, those with and those without hearing loss.

LANGUAGE LEARNING IS COHERENT

The recognition that language learning is coherent, even though children learn language at their own individual paces and in their own individual ways, seems contradictory at first glance. But, when language learning is thought of as a social activity in which each child must work to discover how the people around her or him are using language, it can be understood that children will vary in their rate and style of learning, and that they can be similar generally in working to figure out how language works. Teachers who understand this can allow for a great deal of individuality within a broad general framework which describes their understanding of language learning.

An example provided by Baron (1995, pp. 136-137) describes a kindergarten child who is confused about "they, the, them, and thank." Such a child might decide to pronounce all four words as "they," focusing on the consistent "th" at the beginning of all four words and ignoring at this point the differences in the ends of the words. This represents a temporary solution to the problem of distinguishing among the four words. As long as the teacher can see this as part of an overall and predictable pattern in which each child hypothesizes about language and then continuously tests the hypotheses, the child will be encouraged to continue the hypothesis-testing process. Another child might decide to write all four words using only consonants because at this point he or she has an incomplete understanding of how the vowels work. This child may be confused about the visually similar letters such as *p, b,* and *d* and solve the problem temporarily by pronouncing "tap," " tab," and "tad" in the same way. According to Baron, it is not an inability to distinguish among the letters that is at work when this occurs. Rather, different children need different lengths of time in which to develop the patience to look at all the parts of the word every time in order to identify such words correctly. Some children experiment more than others with language, and how much they experiment can be regarded as simply an individual difference. An accepting environment can make a difference in how much a child experiments. Teachers who criticize and penalize such "wrong" readings may discourage the experimentation that is necessary for the child to figure out the system and thus slow down the progress of the child. Teachers who understand that children can vary widely in their progress to discover how reading works, but that they will use remarkably similar strategies in making the discovery, are more able to take individual needs into account when planning and carrying out instruction. As they work at understanding, children and older students continuously discover processes for setting up and testing hypotheses for how the language system works, as well as content which is stored away in memory because it fits with content stored previously.

Reading and Writing Must Be Meaningful

Teachers who understand the communication process work hard to provide a language-enriched environment by providing many opportunities for speaking, listening, reading, and writing. Hedley and Hedley (1995, p. 16) encourage teachers of children with normal hearing to keep in mind four important points when they decide what and how they will teach their classes. These points are equally important for teachers who have one or more children who are deaf or hard of hearing in class with children with normal hearing:

1. Children can contribute to the development of the curriculum when teachers encourage them to say "I want to know about _____": Teachers who take seriously the need to incorporate children's interests into the class are able to make use of the internal processes described above (memory organized in terms of various schemata stored in meaningful relation to each other, language acquisition regarded as a meaning–making process, etc.)

2. Children should be writing daily about their own topics as well as about topics assigned by the teacher: Practice and feedback about the results of that practice are necessary for the child to make progress in the task of discovering how language works. This means that the teacher must read and respond to the child's writing. Such responses can address both the form and the content of the writing, and which to address will be dependent on the purpose of the assignment.

3. Children should read and listen to a wide variety of poetry, information-
al, and fictional material every day: Learners need models of language
and content and they need a wide variety of them in order to develop the
capacity to understand them and to use them in their own expression.
Classroom activities should include many such opportunities. The child
who is deaf or hard of hearing must be provided the best listening environment possible for listening to the teacher read aloud.

Depending on the child and the situation, this might mean that he or
she sits next to the teacher when the teacher is reading aloud, or it might
mean that the child and teacher use an FM unit so that the sound delivered to the child's ears is as high in quality as possible.

4. Children do better when they have someone who listens — really listens
— to what they say and write: All uses of listening, speaking, reading, and
writing must be for authentic purposes. Each child needs to have meaningful conversations with the teacher and other children as often as possible throughout the school day. These conversations should be about
the content of school work (e.g., a group project or a particular concept), about topics in which the child has interest, and about procedural matters pertinent to making one's way through the school day. This
requires that conversations be related to what the child knows and is
working on and that each person involved in the conversation be careful
to check that understanding occurs at every point in the conversation.

Children should have real writing tasks. "Busywork" or "seatwork" to
which no one responds or to which the teacher responds simply by mark-
ing right and wrong answers is not useful for the learner because the
learner needs a great deal of information about her or his own language
use in order to continue to generate and test hypotheses concerning language. Therefore, the teacher and, at appropriate times, other students
in the class need to be reading what each child writes and responding to
it. "What do you mean by this?" "By that?" "What do you think should
happen next in your story?" "I don't know what this word is. Can you
explain it to me?" "You need the word 'they' here rather than 'them'
because . . ."

This is not to say that there is never a place for some practice on a specific skill. The teacher who has had meaningful interaction with the child
is then in a good position to ask the child to do some meaningful practice. This is different from having the child work through a workbook set
of exercises that may or may not fit the child's needs.

Using Knowledge of What a Good Reader
Does to Individualize Instruction

At this point it is helpful to recall Goodman's description (discussed in Chapter
Two) of what the good reader does (Marzano, 1995, p. 80). The good reader

usually proceeds from left to right and from top to bottom on the page, focusing at strategic places and taking in words and whole phrases at each stop to focus. On the basis of what is seen, the reader creates a meaning by making guesses. These guesses are held tentatively until more reading is done at which time the reader decides whether the guess makes sense or not. If sense has been made, the reader continues; if not, the good reader does some rereading and thinks further about meaning.

Thinking about reading as an interactive process is very useful to the parent, therapist, and teacher of the child who is deaf or hard of hearing. Discovering the child's strengths and weaknesses is the first step in the process of giving individual instruction to the child. While the child who is deaf or hard of hearing may receive individual instruction at school, he or she will need help at home and at therapy sessions as well. The alert adult (the parent, the teacher, the therapist) can observe the child reading and discuss the meaning with her or him in order to figure out what the child is doing when reading. Using strengths to build on weaknesses, the adult can help the child of any age and developmental level to work out a good grasp of the language of the text and how to use it to make meanings.

For example, the beginning reader may know a particular set of words. The adult who knows which words the child knows can help the child choose books to read that contain those words as well as new words. The adult can decide which words will probably be new and present the new words to the child before they begin the reading together. The words known already provide a context for the words that are new, and with practice the new words will soon enter the body of words known by the child. The new words can be taught in a variety of ways, each of which works because of its place in how fluent readers deal with unfamiliar words. Fluent readers make interactive use of many cues and read (1) by sight; (2) by sounding out and blending letters; (3) by analogy to known words; (4) by pronouncing common spelling patterns; and (5) by using context clues (Ehri, 1995, pp. 171-174). All of these ways can be used to help the child learn to recognize the new words a book contains before he or she encounters them in the book.

AN EXAMPLE

Suppose the child has picked out Beverly Cleary's *Ramona the Pest*. The adult can skim through the beginning and decide which words to point out to the child before the child begins to read. Further suppose the adult decides the words are "Ramona Quimby," "Beezus," "Beatrice," "pest," "recently," and "unfair."

The book begins:

"I am not a pest," Ramona Quimby told her big sister Beezus.

"Then stop acting like a pest," said Beezus, whose real name was Beatrice. She was standing by the front window waiting for her friend Mary Jane to walk to school with her.

"I'm not acting like a pest. I'm singing and skipping," said Ramona, who had only recently learned to skip with both feet. Ramona did not think

she was a pest. The people who called her a pest were always bigger and so they could be unfair (pp. 9-10).

First the adult needs to differentiate between words which are probably unknown in speech and words which are known in speech but have not been encountered before in print. Suppose in this case that the child has read other "Ramona" books. He or she may simply need to be reminded of the names "Ramona Quimby," "Beezus," and "Beatrice" because they have been encountered before. This would represent identifying the words *by sight.* These names are unusual enough that they will stand out from the words around them and thus be memorable. They are used frequently which will make it easier for the child to identify them.

"Pest" can be identified by *sounding out and blending letters* because it follows conventional rules of phonics. It has a straightforward pronunciation of "p," a "short e," and a blended "s" and "t." It may not be in the child's listening vocabulary because it may not be used in her or his environment. The adult will need to explain the concept in terms familiar to the child. Perhaps the child has a friend who "pesters" others by patting them on the back to get their attention. Perhaps the child uses "pestering" tactics to get what he or she wants. Using an example and explaining the word by demonstrating endings which can be added to it will help the child along. For example, "Remember the day I said we could go to the playground at 3:00, but you were so excited you couldn't wait? Every 10 minutes you kept reminding me that you wanted to go. You 'pestered' me. You were a 'pest!' Well, Ramona is always excited to do things and her sister calls her a 'pest.'"

"Pest" also rhymes with "best" and can be identified *by analogy to that known word.* "Analogy" is used here to mean "recognizing spelling similarities between new and known words (Ehri, 1995, p. 173)." The adult could write "best" and then cover up the "b" and say, "Let's add a 'p' here at the beginning.

"Recently" can be identified by *pronouncing common spelling patterns.* If the child knows "re" and "ly," which are commonly found in other words, then establishing "cent" is all that needs to be done before putting the three parts of the word together. Possibly, as with "pest," "recently" is a word that represents a concept — as well as a word — that the child does not know. "Remember when we went to the apple orchard to pick apples last weekend?" That wasn't very long ago, so we say we did that "recently."

At the end of the section is "unfair." It can be figured out by using *context clues.* If Ramona thinks that people who call her a pest do it because they are bigger than she is, then the meaning of "unfair" becomes easier to establish. By at the same time combining the knowledge that "un" can be added to the beginning of a word to make it mean the opposite of the original word with knowledge of the sound of "f" and the sight word "air," the child can pronounce the word and put together its meaning in the context.

At this point, the child should be ready to read the beginning of this book, perhaps alone, perhaps with the adult present to help and to enjoy it with the child.

Combining Strategies Is a Strategy

In many cases it is a combination of two or more of the strategies that enables the child to have a meaningful encounter with a new word in a text. This redundancy in language helps in making predictions about meaning: if two or more sources of clues point to a particular pronunciation and a particular meaning, it strengthens the case for accepting that meaning and using it to build further meanings as the reading progresses. What this means in reading is that trying to make meanings by looking at words in isolation does not work because meaning most often depends on words in relation to each other, not on each word by itself.

When Does "Sounding Out" Work?

Keep in mind that word identification strategies work for any reader who already knows the word in speech as long as the visual cues are regular enough for the reader to make a reasonable guess as to how the word sounds. In this case, the reader simply "checks in" to the meaning usually associated with that sound and uses that to make a preliminary guess as to a meaning. One reason reading can be more difficult for the child who is deaf or hard of hearing is that the first encounter with many words will come through reading. For the child with normal hearing, this is not the case; he or she will have *heard* most new reading words before encountering them in print, often in casual or over-heard conversation or by listening to television, and so the child will not need to puzzle over what the words are and what they mean when coming to them in print and using a "sounding out" process. A reader, regardless of whether he or she hears well or not, is not helped by "sounding out" a word he or she does not know, because being able to say the word correctly is not sufficient. "Sounding out" works when the reader figures out a reasonable pronunciation for the unknown visual cues and then matches those sounds to a word in audi-tory memory. Because a reader who is deaf or hard of hearing is likely to know fewer words, he or she will often be at a disadvantage in using this strategy. Therefore, the child who is deaf or hard of hearing needs to be presented very intentionally with more words in speech and needs to have many occasions on which to guess what words mean in context that are followed quickly with appropriate feedback about the suitability of the guess.

Learning to Use Context to Fill in the Gaps

The advice of "talk, talk, talk to your child" holds throughout childhood and adolescence, for this is a good way for new words to be incorporated into her or his working vocabulary so that they are available when encountered in print. Learning to guess what an unknown word means from the context is an extremely valuable skill, one that helps not only in navigating print, but that helps in comprehending what people are saying. The person who is deaf or hard of hearing who learns to get along in the world of people who hear well must fill in gaps when a person's voice drops and a word or phrase is not heard. Being able to fill in that gap by using the context of the surrounding meanings is an extremely useful capability.

Words carry multiple meanings which can cause confusion and create humorous situations. The reader must learn to be on the lookout for such words. *Ramona the Pest* contains such an example in the first chapter. Ramona arrives at school on her first day at kindergarten, and is told by Miss Binney, her teacher, "Sit here for the present (p. 17)." "A present! thought Ramona, and knew at once she was going to like Miss Binney (p. 17)." Ramona has understood the one meaning of "present" that she has in her vocabulary and thinks a gift is on its way. "Nobody had told her she was going to get a present the very first day. What kind of present could it be, she wondered, trying to remember if Beezus had ever been given a present by her teacher (p. 17)." When Miss Binney shows Howie, Ramona's friend to his seat, she says, "Howie, I would like you to sit here (p. 17)." Ramona's thoughts race as she listens carefully to what Miss Binney says to each child. When Miss Binney does not mention a present to anyone else, Ramona concludes that she has been singled out to receive a special gift, and she speculates about what it will be and how it will be wrapped. It is not until Ramona refuses to leave her seat for an activity that the teacher discovers that Ramona has misunderstood her words and gently explains to her, "You see 'for the present' means for now. I meant that I wanted you to sit here for now because later I may have the children sit at different desks (p. 27)." By this time the reader has been entertained by Ramona's quite logical and understandable mistake. The reader who does not know that words can have more than one meaning can learn about this phenomenon from this example. And the adult reading this book with a child can learn a great deal about how children constantly have to figure out what is going on in their world as new activities and words come at them.

Purposes for Reading

Sometimes children misconstrue the purpose for reading and understand it to be one of pronouncing words correctly. When done in meaningful contexts, reading has at least three purposes, at least one of which can apply to the reading of any text: (1) vicarious experience and enjoyment; (2) gaining new information; and (3) validating what one thinks he or she knows (Marzano, p. 81). Teachers and parents can help children and adolescents find meaning in their reading by helping them establish good reasons and purposes before beginning the reading of a particular piece. Such purposes must go beyond that of doing some reading simply because the teacher made an assignment. The adult can help the child and the adolescent engage in the necessary purpose setting by helping her or him ask questions before, during, and after reading.

Vicarious experience and enjoyment are powerful reasons to read. No one can experience everything, and reading lets us see what it's like to climb Mount

Everest and swim the English Channel. It also helps us to understand how we feel about something and to compare our feelings with those of others. Vicarious experience and enjoyment questions include: Have I ever done anything like this? Felt this way? Thought this way? How are my experiences similar and different to these characters? Does this story help me understand something going on in my life? What do I like and dislike about this story? Why?

Information gathering is another powerful reason to read. Remembering facts about the world around us can be helpful in getting along day to day. Learning where to find certain kinds of facts is the mark of an educated person. Information gathering questions can include: Is this information useful? Does it help my project? What other kinds of information do I need to locate?

Validation questions make our inquiry more complex. Being able to evaluate what we encounter is regarded by most as one of the highest level skills (Bloom, 1956). Learning to do it can begin very early with the young reader gradually learning to take a critical look at the meaning he or she is creating during reading. Validation questions could include: Does this information agree or disagree with what I have already learned or found in another source? Do I need to look further for more support for this information? Older readers can begin setting the standard for evidence by asking: What constitutes evidence I will accept? Where is the proof?

The process of reading for meaning is a gradual one of the adult helping the child in these ways until the child can ask these kinds of questions independently without being prompted. Note that the questions can be asked at any grade level and that they span reading materials from stories to nonfiction accounts.

Using Knowledge of What a Good Writer Does to Individualize Instruction

Good writers work hard at writing. Their words do not flow onto the page in full well-formed sentences. Most writers compose within a cycle which includes prewriting, writing, rewriting, and editing stages (Smith, 1982, pp. 103-137).

During prewriting the writer thinks about what he or she wants to say. This may involve making notes or lists or doing what is called "freewriting," which is simply writing down all one's thoughts as they occur. Each of these processes is performed in order to capture the preliminary possibilities for the work on paper. At this stage the writer is not expected to write in good form, nor must the writer like or want to use all the ideas that emerge. This stage is simply preliminary, and it may appear to be messy and disorganized.

When the writer is ready to write, he or she chooses from the ideas, words, and phrases generated in prewriting and makes a plan for the work to follow. In formal terms this might be an outline; less formally, the plan may be a simple list to follow during the writing so that important points are not left out. The writer begins writing about each element in the outline or list, paying some but not total attention to the form of the words and phrases.

When the writer feels satisfied that he or she has fulfilled the goal of writing about everything on the list, the work is set aside for a time in order to get some distance from it. This may be a few minutes, a few hours, or even days depending on the work and the purposes for it. When the writer returns to it, rewriting begins. The writer reads the work carefully and may ask one or more others to read it, as well. Writing groups in school function to provide readers for each writer's work, and it is common to see children sitting together reading each other's papers and giving each other reactions and suggestions about them. On the basis of what the writer thinks about changing the writing, the writer begins to revise the writing, adding here and taking away there until he or she feels some satisfaction that the piece says what he or she wants it to say.

The final stage is editing. In this stage the writer looks carefully at the work, making sure that spelling is correct and that words are used appropriately. It can be difficult to find mistakes because involvement in the meaning of one's own writing can cause one's mistakes to become invisible. For this reason, children often help each other in this phase as part of school writing groups.

At times all of the elements of the writing cycle are brought in at the level of writing one sentence; the steps need not be followed only on the piece as a whole. Adults trying to help children learn to write can do so by paying attention to the need for the steps and not expecting perfection immediately. Receiving individual help from adults who remember that writing is a process of discovering meaning and putting it into words helps children become good writers at all levels.

Frequent Reading Leads to Good Writing

The child who is deaf or hard of hearing benefits from frequent exposure to well-formed written language because the conventions of language, including spelling, are repeatedly available as models to her or him. Avid readers, regardless of their hearing abilities, expose themselves to more models of written language and are more likely to be good writers than people who do not read often, though good reading ability does not guarantee good spelling ability. Much can be learned about patterns of words and conventional uses of words through repeated encounters with written language. I have had the feeling in talking with well-read people, those with and those without deafness, that I am talking with a person who is so articulate that he or she "sounds like a book." These are people who have taken their predominant language patterns from the reading they have done. These patterns show up in their writing, as well. As I followed Annie's writing through high school, I noticed a real shift in her writing voice as she began to read more adult material.

Spelling is usually easier for children and adults who read frequently and who read for meaning, because words which carry similar meanings have similar spelling features. The words "medicine" and "medical" have "medic" in common, and "medic" suggests something about the meaning of each word. If each were spelled the way it is pronounced, we would have "medisin" and "medikal," which would not provide clues as to their common root meaning (Smith, 1978, p. 143). If one tries to write exactly what one hears, it can be hard to spell correctly, and it is especially difficult to write a word that does not follow conventional spelling rules (try spelling "hors d'oeuvres" that way!). The child who is deaf or hard of hearing can use her or his visual abilities coupled with her or his growing ability to fill in the gaps left by unheard words. These are real strengths the child can build on in order to take in the language cues through print, cues that children with normal hearing get through casual listening.

Establishing a "Thinking Environment"

As I have tried to explain, reading and writing are both thinking processes which are best nurtured in what Bernhardt and Antonacci (1995, pp. 244-247) term a "thinking environment." Children learn to think about and use language whether it is spoken or written and whether they are producing it (speaking or writing) or receiving it (listening or reading) by being in such an environment.

A thinking environment provides:

1. *Many kinds of texts to read and to write:*
   Learners should be encouraged to make choices about what they will read and write. Adults can best nurture children during their choosing by being alert to each child's interests and making sure there are reading materials and writing possibilities available that fit those interests. In part this works because the learner has internalized the requisite words and meanings about the given interest in order to read, write, and think about that subject area. This is especially important for children with hearing impairment because their vocabularies are usually not developed evenly across subject areas. In the process of working from a strength, the child will add to her or his vocabulary in ways that will enable her or him to understand language used in other areas. Each child determines by her or his interests what materials are special to her or him, so the question of having the "correct" materials begins to disappear. What is vital is to have a variety of materials readily available to each child. Encouraging use of the school and public libraries helps in reaching this goal.

2. *Interaction between students and teachers in reading and writing texts:*
   Reading and writing are enriched through opportunities to talk with someone else about one's thinking. Such talk gives children chances to compare interpretations with each other and with an adult. A discussion of even slightly different interpretations is far more interesting and enlightening than feedback from a teacher concerning right and wrong answers on a worksheet. Sharing their writing gives children chances to find out how someone else understood it, which helps them shape their revisions as they strive to communicate. All such meaningful talk helps

build vocabulary, use of conventional grammar and word order, fluency, and articulation in all children, but especially in children who are deaf or hard of hearing.

3. *Involvement:*

Involvement includes the interactions the learner can have with materials as well as with others in the thinking environment. Involvement presses learners to think in more complex ways and to add to their ways of looking at their worlds and usually results when children are reading, writing, and talking about ideas and information that they find interesting. The child with hearing impairment can feel isolated from others because he or she cannot always pick up on surrounding casual conversation, so providing for and expecting involvement is particularly helpful to her or him. In addition, the child who is deaf or hard of hearing has an easier time when the subject is defined because then the vocabulary with which to deal with it is at least in part defined.

4. *Realistic expectation of success:*

When the adult in the environment expects success, the learners do, also, and they will strive to achieve it. It is entirely realistic to expect success. At times, however, the adult expects success to be achieved according to an unrealistic timetable. It is better to find suitable ways to support the learner and, thus, nurture achievement than to declare failure in some area when a certain level of achievement has not been reached by a specified time. Children who are deaf or hard of hearing may need more time, but that does not mean they cannot be successful.

5. *Learning to take responsibility for one's learning:*

Children who feel they are thinking for themselves rather than for someone else are more likely to learn with purpose and thus learn more. In the case of the child who is deaf or hard of hearing, it is easy for the adult to excuse the child for not paying attention and not putting forth effort. Becoming accountable for listening and learning through listening, reading, and writing gives the child who is deaf or hard of hearing evidence of her or his abilities and adds to self-esteem.

6. *Opportunities for practice:*

As with any other endeavor, thinking requires practice. Practice in thinking is enhanced by frequent communication with others through speaking, listening, reading, and writing. The child who is deaf or hard of hearing needs more such opportunities than the child with normal hearing because of the gaps he or she has in language achievement. These gaps cannot be closed without extensive practice with people who use language in fluent and conventional ways.

7. *Encouragement for risk-taking without condemnation for mistakes:*
All learners need to feel they can try something without fear of condemnation for mistakes. After all, there would be no new discoveries if people could not experiment. Children are often compared to scientists (Ruddell & Ruddell, 1994, p. 83) as they figure out how things in their world work, including language. Helping children understand that they can think about and learn from their mistakes helps them become less fearful of making mistakes and makes them feel secure enough to take each new step. For the child who is deaf or hard of hearing, such encouragement is particularly helpful because he or she is more often in the position of having to guess and thus take risks than is the child with normal hearing.

8. *Help from a teacher who gives positive feedback rather than negative judgment:*
Thinking thrives in environments where learners are shown what is working well in their thought processes. The adult who points out and praises successes is in a better position to offer corrective and constructive criticism when it is necessary. Finding strengths and helping the child use them to eliminate weaknesses adds to self-esteem by using knowledge that the learner already has, which is a more efficient way of learning. Children with hearing impairment may feel less equipped than children with normal hearing, and so they especially are in need of positive feedback.

7

What Other Questions Are Parents, Therapists, and Teachers Asking?

Highlights

▼ Good readers fill in gaps they encounter by using their background knowledge.

▼ There are normal progressions of language learning, and children who are deaf or hard of hearing often follow them.

▼ Using words in conventional ways is more important than pronouncing them in conventional ways.

▼ Sign language is a special and well-formed language that is distinctly different from written language.

▼ Good teaching about a wide variety of subjects helps children take proficiency tests.

▼ Young children need help and role models in learning how to use books.

▼ Just as any child could have Attention Deficit Disorder (ADD), so could the child who is deaf or hard of hearing.

▼ Adults need to help children see reading as fun and important.

▼ The team working with the child can best decide together what kind of help the child needs.

▼ The purpose of both formal and informal assessment is to make instructional decisions.

▼ Some children begin reading by identifying whole words, others begin by identifying individual letters, and still others by doing both.

▼ Knowledge of the language that is to be read is necessary for learning how to read.

▼ Techniques for helping the child who is deaf or hard of hearing as well as learning disabled are the same as those for children with normal hearing and learning disabilities.

▼ Teamwork is necessary among the adults who work with and care for the child.

▼ Computer technology can be helpful but cannot substitute for human interaction.

▼ Children can learn to use conventional language as one part of the writing process.

I COLLECTED THE FOLLOWING QUESTIONS FROM PARENTS, THERAPISTS, AND teachers at the Auditory Verbal International conference in Cuyahoga Falls, Ohio, in July of 1995.

1. Can written language and reading surpass the child's spoken language level?

There is a sense in which this appears to be possible because, as the child becomes more proficient at using language, he or she uses language in its various forms to learn more about language and all its possibilities. This process is, of course, not limited to children; it is learned in childhood and continues throughout life, and it accounts for how we learn new information from reading and listening to others. For the person who is deaf or hard of hearing, written language offers the advantage of staying put indefinitely so that it can be studied and thought about. It does not disappear as spoken words do, and all the words are visible, whereas in spoken language some words can be missed because they are not detectable by the ears. The gaps in written text that can cause comprehension problems are gaps in knowledge of the language (word order, usage, individual word meanings, etc.), and these gaps can be bridged by asking questions, consulting a dictionary, and doing some strategic guessing. For the person who is deaf or hard of hearing, then, written language (both the writing and the reading of it) can serve as a very powerful way of receiving and sending information, and it can appear that the person knows more written language than spoken language simply because the written language can be processed more readily in certain circumstances.

What must always be kept in mind, though, are the relationships between and among the various ways of using language. Some parents, teachers, and therapists have been persuaded that the child who is deaf or hard of hearing cannot learn spoken language, and they have decided to concentrate on written language, instead. This thinking is flawed, because spoken language and its social roots (Vygotsky, 1992) are the beginning and, therefore, the foundation for all other language uses. In a person who is learning, there is a continuous spiral of language achievement. As the learner increases knowledge of each form of language, he or she is in a better position to develop a better grasp of the other forms. Neglecting any one of the forms makes it more difficult to make progress in the others. This is not to overlook the phenomenon that for some people, whether or not their hearing is normal, reading and writing are easier than speaking; for others, it is the opposite. This is due, simply, to individual differences in learning and communication styles.

2. Is there a timeline of expectations for emergence, production of morphemes, syntax, etc.?

Agnes Ling has published *Schedules of Development in Audition, Speech, Language, and Communication for Hearing Impaired Infants and their Families* (1977), which lays out the progression of such development in the following areas: Audition, Speech, Language, and Communication. This appears in a small booklet designed as a series of checklists which can be helpful in deciding what to present next.

My experience in trying to chart Annie's developing language was that it was fairly easy to do at the beginning when she did not have much language. I gave up on the task after a sudden explosion of words began to come out of her, and I could no longer keep up.

3. During reading, should we constantly correct the speech of mispronounced words? Should we do so when the child is speaking?

For several reasons, constant correction of the child's speech in either case is not a good idea. Such correction may give the child the idea that it is the production of sound that is important rather than the creation of meaning. Children with normal hearing sometimes get this idea which brings them to the conclusion that reading is a performance rather than a way to get some new information or to enjoy a story. Their attention goes to the performance rather than to any generation of meaning, and they have difficulty making progress in making sense of reading. I have heard enough children with normal hearing "read" a page of text, with almost perfect pronunciation, only to find that they have comprehended almost nothing of the story, to know that good pronunciation is not evidence of good reading. This phenomenon could become even more extreme in the child who is deaf or hard of hearing if he or she is operating with more than usual confusion about how to use words to communicate with others. On the other hand I have heard enough children, with and without deafness, read aloud with a number of mispronunciations and even incorrect word identifications to know that it is possible for them to get a general idea of the text despite their errors.

Constant correction also gets in the way of the thought processes necessary for putting together the ideas and meanings suggested by the words of the text.

Each correction serves as an interruption during which whatever is in short term memory fades away. It is necessary for any one of us to have a flow of ideas through short term memory in order to think about something. When such thinking is interrupted and blocked out, we must start our thinking over again, which prevents us from creating a chain of ideas that relate to each other. This holds true for children who hear well and children who do not.

Another drawback of constant — or even frequent — correction is that the child can lose confidence in her or himself as a learner. Imagine how you would feel doing your job if you were corrected at every turn! The attentive adult is in a position to choose reading materials that provide the right amount of challenge so that the emerging reader can have the feelings of accomplishment that accompany learning something new.

This is not to say that pronunciation and word identification are not important. Of course they are. This leads us to the question of when and how to help the child pronounce and identify words in conventional ways. At this point I want to point out that the "correct" pronunciation of many English words varies from country to country and from region to region in different parts of the United States. At very least this is what we call "having an accent" or "speaking in another dialect." Most people think that other people have accents and dialects and that they themselves do not, when, in fact, everyone speaks with an accent and in a particular dialect. Think about how you pronounce "New Orleans" compared to the way a U.S. northerner and a U.S. southerner does, or the way you pronounce "about" compared to the way a citizen of the United States and a citizen of Canada does, and you will have some idea of this. With a little thought you can generate numerous examples of differences in speech patterns. I bring this up to underline the fact that in working with any child you need to be aware that you are teaching her or him the conventional ways of speaking in your environment.

My experience is that, especially during the early years, the best way to teach about pronunciation is apart from teaching about comprehension of what one is reading. Doing some preparation before asking the child to read aloud helps the child become more confident about reading aloud. It is difficult to read anything aloud before having read it silently. Even proficient adult readers like to read something silently before going public with it. We usually ask children to read aloud so that we can get some insight into what they are doing when they are reading. When they get stuck on a particular word, then we know that we need to work on that word. When they look puzzled at a certain point, we know that we need to give an explanation. We can ask the child to look over the words of the text or to read it silently first and to tell us if there are any parts that he or she needs help with. Then we can help the child rehearse certain words before reading aloud. We can also talk about what they mean and how the child can relate them to experiences he or she has had. (Oh, yes, that word is "_____." It's like _____ that you already know from the book about _____. See how they have the same ending?)

Reading *can* be used intentionally to work on pronunciation, though. When that is your intent, you must explain to the child that that is what you want to work on for a particular time period. You can take real advantage of the fact that written language, despite its many irregularities, has enough regularities that the letters can show the child who is deaf or hard of hearing where certain sounds are. For example, Annie had difficulty hearing the letter "s" because her particular hearing loss prevented her from hearing high frequency sounds unless she was in very good listening conditions. (With the cochlear implant, she is now able to hear frequencies she never heard before.) Because it is very difficult to pronounce what one doesn't hear, as a young child Annie did not know that many words had "s's" in them until she began to learn to read. We did not begin concentrating on such articulation, though, until she was 7 or 8 years old, even though she had begun to learn to read when she was about 4.

One exercise that was very helpful to her involved having her read a funny story I had written that contained many words with "s's" in it. I told her ahead of time that I wanted her to read it out loud to practice the "s" sounds and to pay attention to where the "s's" were in the words. Then it was easy to point out where she was putting the "s" in appropriately and where she was leaving it out inappropriately. I would also ask her to read other pieces aloud and say that I wanted her to see if she could pronounce 25 words with "s" sounds correctly. Then I would count on my fingers, holding one up for each correct "s" as she read, or I would tally them on paper, stopping and congratulating her when she reached the goal. Pronouncing "s" was so hard for her that another approach of ours was to give her a necklace (which has an "s" sound in it!) that we called her "s" necklace. I suggested that she touch the necklace to remind herself to pay attention to the words she knew that had "s's" in them and to be careful to say the "s" when she said the word. One could do these sorts of exercises with other sound-to-letter relationships that a particular child needs help with.

As for telling the reader words that he or she encounters in reading either orally or silently, I would let the situation dictate whether to simply provide the word or whether to help the child discover what the word is. A child who is exhibiting frustration should be told what the word is and perhaps be given an explanation of some sort. If the child does not seem to be frustrated, the adult can ask the child what kind of word would fit the meaning, and quite often the child can guess what the word is *if the word is already in the child's speaking vocabulary*. If the adult knows that the child has just seen the word on a previous page, he or she can prompt the child with clues associated with the meaning or can point out the word where it appeared earlier. Perhaps the word shares some features with a word already known. The adult can point that out to help the child guess.

A good rule of thumb to follow is that if there are more than about five words on a page that the child in the beginning stages of reading does not know, then that particular text is probably too hard for the child at that point because it presents too many gaps in meaning. More attention needs to be given to the new concepts and the words associated with them before the child will be able to read that particular text fluently. If the text holds great interest for the child, then he or she will have great incentive to learn the new words and concepts, and so the adult and the child can proceed together with it. If not, then trying to read the text will produce a great deal of frustration. While some children deal with frustration better than others, it is usually better to avoid it when possible.

4. How can I expect my child to learn English reading and writing if he or she is using sign language?

English and American Sign Language (ASL) are two different languages, and so you cannot expect the child who signs ASL, but who does not know spoken English to learn to read and write English very easily. ASL is a three-dimensional, visual language that is not spoken. English is spoken and heard, and in general requires listening in order to learn it. The important factor to take into account is that a child cannot learn to read a language in which he or she does not already know how to communicate. I have been told that Signing Exact English is cumbersome, but a child who knows that would have a better chance of learning to read some English because he or she would already know English word order. Bypassing the spoken word does not work in English, because, however irregular the language is in its sound-to-letter relationships, those relationships serve as powerful links that help the language user generate and read a countless number of original statements. A language such as Chinese works from pictures that represent meanings, and so different dialects have different sounds and words for the characters. This enables people who know the characters to read the writing of people who speak very differently from them, but it does not enable them to understand each other in speaking (Samuels, 1994, p. 375). ASL functions to some extent in that same way for language users from different areas, but that dialect feature does not aid in the reading of English. Higher achievement in reading for both individuals who are deaf or hard of hearing and those with normal hearing is associated with higher achievement in knowing the spoken language and how most speakers and readers of the language use it.

5. How can I prepare children to pass state competency tests?

As more and more states are requiring the passing of competency tests, this question is being asked for all children, those who are deaf or hard of hearing and those with normal hearing alike. All children should receive pertinent instruction about how to take such tests so that they understand how the tests "work," however, some programs are spending a great deal of time teaching children test-wise behaviors that help them become better guessers on such tests. This bothers me because then the test score will not reflect the child's achievement in the content or process area; rather it reflects an ability to guess well. Instead, I believe that parents, teachers, and therapists should work to prepare children to read, write, speak, listen, and think to the best of their abilities and then the test will take care of itself. Nothing special needs to be done except to try to ensure that the child is making progress in learning in relation to other children in the same setting. Test results should be used to make instructional decisions, and so people should ask for as much explanation of scores and purposes of the tests as possible in order to know in what areas to help the child. Children who are deaf or hard of hearing who process language more slowly than children with normal hearing should be allowed to have more time to take such tests.

6. What do you do with the child who just wants to turn the pages?

The child who "just wants to turn the pages" is quite likely exhibiting some knowledge about how books work, so this is a good sign. This child may be experimenting with reading behaviors he or she has seen in others. Sitting down with the child to look at picture books together, allowing her or him to turn the pages would encourage the behavior and put it in a positive setting. Asking the child to turn the pages when the adult is reading aloud to her or him would do the same. Assuming the child is just refusing to pay attention is usually non-productive and should be avoided. Instead, the adult can try to find out what is motivating the child's behavior.

Marie Clay has developed a measure called "Concepts About Print" that can be used to compile information about the child's understanding of how books work.

> *The teacher says, "I'll read this book. You help me." And then he or she asks the child to do things such as, "Show me where I start reading. Which way do I go? Where do I go after that? Point to the words while I read"* (Lyons et al., 1993, p. 10).

It could be that the child in question has little understanding of how books work and simply needs to be read to more so that he or she has more experience with words and books. It could be that the child's language abilities are not yet formed to the extent that listening to a book makes sense to her or him. This does not mean, however, that the adult should stop reading to the child and wait until language abilities catch up. Reading to the child is one part of helping the language abilities catch up.

If the child in question is in the early part of kindergarten or younger, he or she is not unusual in comparison with children with normal hearing. In a study of 141 kindergartners in Columbus, Ohio, the average child knew only 4 of 24 concepts about print that were evaluated. The average child could hold the book right-side up and understood that books are read left-to-right and top-to-bottom, but could not read the words or match printed words to the spoken words of the adult reader. By the end of kindergarten, the average child knew about 50 upper and lower case letters and had acquired 13 or 14 of the 24 concepts about print (Lyons et al., 1993, p. 112). More can be found about Clay's "Concepts About Print" in Clay (1989).

7. Could the child who is deaf or hard of hearing also have Attention Deficit Disorder (ADD)?

ADD or ADHD (Attention Deficit Hyperactivity Disorder) is a possibility for any child, the child who is deaf or hard of hearing included, though it is estimated that only 3% to 5% of school-age children have the disorder (Berk, L., 1994, p. 279). The symptoms can range from mild to severe, so some children who have trouble concentrating are possibly not diagnosed. That only a small number of children have ADD or ADHD is no consolation when faced with the possibility that yours does. Children with the disorder are often inattentive, impulsive, and easily frustrated. They may or may not also be far more active than average children. Parents, therapists, and teachers can help such children by structuring lessons so that short work sessions and time to get up and move around are alternated. Children who are deaf or hard of hearing often exhibit ADD- or ADHD-like symptoms, because they are not "tuning in" to the world around them. More attention to helping the child learn to listen will help, though; children taught through the Auditory-Verbal approach usually develop great ability to concentrate. The ability to sustain attention grows in the developing person, so adult attention spans are longer than children's. Sometimes adults think children have trouble paying attention when they are really asking for too long a period of paying attention for a young child who is simply exhibiting a normal attention span. Parents who suspect their child has ADD or ADHD should seek testing from a psychologist experienced in diagnosing them and dealing with the problems they cause.

8. How do you motivate a child to take time to read a book (without taking control of the book)?

Children need to see reading as fun and important. They can learn this easily by seeing the adults and older children in their lives reading frequently. Furthermore, making time for communicating puts the stamp of importance on communication activities. Less access to television, videos, and video games provides more time for speaking, listening, reading, writing, and thinking, and that is the best reason I can think of to seek a balance in their use for all children. Most young children would rather have the attention of a "real-life" adult than watch a medium where interaction is not possible. If we want a child to learn to read and to value reading, then setting aside time for reading with the child is imperative. The bedtime reading routine is a tradition that builds readers and simultaneously builds closeness between adult and child. As children grow older, it is tempting to stop reading with them and to simply expect that they will read on their own. In cases where this does not happen, the adults in the child's life need to analyze what is going on in the situation. Are the adults in the child's life setting a good example by reading and talking about what they read with real interest? Are there books, magazines, and newspapers readily available in the house? Are the adults making meaningful and pleasant time to sit down with the child to read? Are the adults taking the child to the library so that he or she can pick out books that are of interest? It is not likely that a child who does not see reading going on in the lives of people he respects will read on her or his own. It is never too late to resume or to start reading with or to a child, because we are never too old to be read to. That interpersonal connection in the process of communication is vital; otherwise people would not flock to hear authors of books read their works and to have their books signed. An older child who is not reading on her or his own may still be struggling with trying to decipher the system and may need more help to become an independent reader. This can be discovered through the process of reading with the child, and then help can be sought.

9. How do you know if your child who is deaf or hard of hearing requires professional help in reading and writing? What should you look out for?

Children learn about reading and writing from a variety of sources, because, as Britton (1993) makes clear, the task of learning language and how to read and write it is one of discovering the ways people use language in communicating with one another. Therefore, the adult in the child's life should be alert to what the child does in the presence of print material (books, magazines, cereal boxes, fun-meal containers, etc.), crayons, pencils, and paper. The adult who is paying attention can figure out what the child thinks the purposes of all of those things are. Does the child turn the pages one-by-one working from front to back? Does he or she pay attention to the eye-catching games on cereal boxes? Does he or she ask "What does this say?" Does he or she write and draw pictures and seem to enjoy creating with crayons and pencils? These are sample questions to pose as the reading and writing processes are in their beginning stages. Parents and therapists of young children who are deaf or hard of hearing can think of their work in the area of literacy development as that of trying to deliver a child who is ready to learn more about reading and writing to the kindergarten or first grade teacher. Therefore, if the child is not showing any particular interest in written symbols or in making marks of some sort on paper, the adult should be seeking out ways of introducing the child to these processes, not through using formal instruction, but through informal ways such as reading aloud to the child, pointing out what various words and symbols "say," and being sure to use reading and writing in the presence of the child.

In years past, educators tried to designate a certain age when reading and writing instruction should begin and some even gave the advice to parents to leave all teaching about literacy to the schools. Current understanding about how all the communication processes interrelate considers the learning of literacy to be a process that unfolds over a period of time beginning in infancy and ending in adulthood, so it is necessary that parents and others important to the child be involved. The best kind of adult involvement appears now to be that of creating an environment enriched by emphasis on language and all its many uses.

In discussing reading readiness, Delores Durkin (1987, pp. 57-89) makes the point that the child's readiness for formal reading instruction must be seen in relation to the methods and goals of each type of formal reading instruction. This means that some children arrive at school and find instruction that fits them and others do not. Parents, and especially the parent(s) of a child who is deaf or hard of hearing, need to be talking with the teachers throughout the year and using a team approach (parent, teacher, therapist, special needs teacher, itinerant teacher of children who are deaf or hard of hearing, etc.) so that they can determine whether the instruction is fitting the child's particular needs. Each teacher and specialist on the team is a professional, but it must be understood that professionals can disagree about methods and approaches. This is where the parent must listen with openness and flexibility, because it will not be unusual to get a variety of opinions, each coming from a different professional orientation and preparation. The task of the parent is to attempt to sort out the advice when it conflicts and to seek the best learning environment for the child.

The parent should talk with the teacher(s) and principal of the school, and together they should decide which programs of the school are appropriate for the child. *Reading Recovery,* which I describe below, is one example of a successful approach to helping children in the early grades who are not making suitable progress in reading. It is widely known and practiced, but is not in use everywhere. Parents should consider its relevant aspects in evaluating the approach offered by their child's school. It is important to remember there is no "magic cure" in the form of the perfect program for dealing with every child's reading difficulties.

In *Reading Recovery,* children are taken through activities that usually yield interest in and readiness for reading. Each child in *Reading Recovery* participates in a 30-minute per day one-to-one relationship with a teacher during which "the teacher provides just enough support to help the child accomplish tasks that will lead to learning (Lyons et al., 1993, p. 8). Note that *Reading Recovery* does not involve "skill and drill," but instead builds on the knowledge about language that each child brings to each session. *Reading Recovery* is, however, intensive. Its goal is to help the child catch up to the curriculum being presented in the regular classroom, and so children are not taken out of the usual instructional activities in that classroom. *Reading Recovery* is regarded as "something extra" (Lyons et al., 1993, p. 5) which helps the child overcome the effects of a slow start.

In a typical 30-minute *Reading Recovery* session there are four parts: reading familiar books; recording a running record of yesterday's new book; writing; and introduction and first reading of a new book (Lyons et al., 1993, pp. 5-7). Throughout the session the teacher takes great care in observing the child's strategies for reading and writing in an effort to understand how the child understands the process so that he or she can give feedback to the child and help the process along. The first step, reading familiar books, involves the child's favorite books from which he or she chooses one or several to read to the teacher. The teacher comments and gives help where needed, even reading along with the child when necessary. Next, the child reads from yesterday's new book with the teacher making notes about the child's reading behaviors from which to make instructional decisions. Some instructional decisions are made and acted upon during the reading; others are saved for later. Third, the child gets to write during each session in small books constructed from ordinary paper. The top half of each page is used for experimenting and learning to form certain letters and words. The bottom half is used for the child's message. This is something like the language experience book I described in chapter four. Words in the bottom half are spelled conventionally, as each will be used for future reading practice, and so the teacher gives help where necessary to accomplish this. The sentences are written also on sentence strips so that the words can be cut apart and assembled in many different ways. Last, the teacher presents the child with a new book to read. The teacher chooses this book because it contains something that will challenge and stretch the child's reading abilities, but it will not be so challenging as to be overwhelming.

Sessions continue until the child has caught up with the class in reading and writing.

10. What assessment tools can be used?

Assessment can be a difficult matter. Parents should be involved in assessment done in the school and during therapy. They should ask as many questions as necessary to find out what is being assessed each time and how the outcome of each assessment will be used in the child's education. Sometimes parents ask whether this test or that test is "good" or not. The answer always depends on the purposes for using an assessment tool, the conditions under which it is administered, and the quality of the information it yields in terms of decisions that can be made from such information.

Assessments are categorized as standardized and as informal. Standardized tests are published by test-making companies and usually serve to compare an individual child to a very large sample of children from across the country. Informal tests are usually teacher-made tests which are designed to enable the teacher to observe the child's interactions with certain materials.

Standardized paper and pencil tests may yield results that appear to tell us something, when in reality the poor scores could be demonstrating the child's misunderstanding of the directions, boredom with the task and content, lack of background knowledge, or something else altogether. This is why assessment of a child's achievement should include many examples of the child's performance representing a variety of literacy tasks. Each portion of the assessment is but a small piece in an overall description of the child's strengths and challenges; it is the pattern of achievement that is important. A score on a standardized test is limited in many ways and should always be considered in the context of other examples of the child's work. Each standardized test score will vary depending on the interest the child has in the subject matter used in the test, how the child felt while taking the test (hungry? anxious?), and to what extent the test fits what the child has been learning. Therefore, standardized test scores are not absolutely accurate measures of the child's achievement.

Teachers can use an Informal Reading Inventory (IRI) to try to get an idea of how the child is approaching reading and how much of the process he or she has learned to use. The typical IRI makes use of a series of paragraphs which get progressively more difficult. The child reads the paragraphs in order for the teacher and answers questions the teachers asks. Throughout the inventory, the teacher listens and records what the child reads correctly and incorrectly. The record then guides the teacher in making instructional decisions for the child.

Assessment should always have the goal of helping the teacher fit instruction to the child's needs rather than labeling the child as a high or low achiever. Therefore, the assessment that yields a richer description of the child's abilities and weaknesses is more valuable than one that simply yields a number or cluster of numbers. For this reason, a portfolio approach to assessment is becoming more widely used. In this approach, the child (supervised by the teacher) collects work he or she has done and puts it together in a folder or box so that the range of the child's responses in a variety of circumstances can be seen easily.

11. What do you do when your child is interested in letters and words but has not had much practice in connecting sounds and letters?

The adult should attend to that interest, as it signals the beginnings of reading and writing. While there appear to be some "symptoms" of being ready to read (ability to identify letters and their sounds, fondness for books and stories, ability to sit still long enough to page through a book, etc.), learning the letters and sounds is not necessarily the beginning. Some children begin by identifying whole words as they have learned to match them up with what the person reading to them says. Some begin by identifying symbols for products and stores. Others seem to benefit from learning the names and sounds of the letters. There are many routes into reading and writing. The best thing to do is to pay attention to the way the child is responding to print and symbols and help the child do more of whatever he or she has already begun to do.

12. How is it best to proceed teaching reading/writing to a child who exhibits the "normal" reading readiness/writing skills of a 4- to 5-year-old, but the child's language and vocabulary are severely delayed? Or should you proceed?

The child whose language and vocabulary are severely delayed is not exhibiting reading readiness. Because one must know and be able to use the language that is to be read, the best way to work with such a child is to concentrate on her or his acquisition of language and vocabulary. Using a language experience book can help with this. Reading aloud with the child and playing all sorts of games that use language can, too. Above all, putting extra effort into language and speech therapy and creating a language-enriched environment are essential at this time. This is not to say that the child should be kept from books, magazines, and other chances to read. All such opportunities should also be available to the child. But, the child whose language and vocabulary are severely delayed needs other formal and informal instruction more than he or she needs reading instruction.

13. What if the child who is deaf or hard of hearing also has learning disabilities?

True learning disabilities are processing problems associated with "a significant discrepancy between IQ and achievement caused by problems in such basic psychological processes as remembering or perceiving" (Lefrancois, 1991, pp. 274-275). In the case of the child who is deaf or hard of hearing, it is difficult to sort out what part of an observed deficiency is caused by the hearing loss and what part is caused by a learning disability. While there are no magic cures for learning disabilities, there are approaches whose goal is to equip the learning disabled person with strategies by which to compensate for the learning disability. When a learning disability is suspected, the child's learning behaviors and problems should be evaluated by a competent specialist who can guide the parents, therapist, and teachers in tailoring their approach to the child's specific needs, just as would be done for the child with normal hearing.

14. How can parents work with teachers? Teachers with parents? Therapists?

Parents, teachers, and therapists need to see themselves operating as a team working toward the best for the child. This means that each person on the team must respect the needs, questions, fears, and ideas of the others on the team. Communication between and among the members of the team is essential and all must guard against being less than open with one another. There is always the danger that two on such a team will "gang up" against another, tallying up hurts and offenses "caused" by the other side. A moment or two of reflection will quickly demonstrate that this will not be in the best interest of the child. Communication can take the form of notes, memos, meetings, and attendance in each other's spheres. It's a good idea, periodically, for the parent to see the therapist and the teacher working with the child, for the therapist to visit home and school, and for the teacher to visit home and therapy.

It is possible for members of the team to hold differing philosophies about what to do with the child. As long as they are not profoundly in opposition to each other, the parent can probably learn from both and help the child do so as well. When there is too wide a difference, though, the parent will need to make decisions which could result in a new team. This could mean changing schools or changing therapists.

15. How is computer technology best used for teaching reading and writing?

Learning keyboarding and using a computer for word processing are a lot of fun for many children, and ability in this area will help in the long run in school and other learning. However, I do not recommend "workbook" drills on the computer as some magic fix, even though computer effects and rewards are more fun than what a paper workbook can do. The problem is that the "workbook drill and skill" approach, whether delivered electronically or on paper, does not require much interaction or much thinking, both of which usually require using language. For the child who is deaf or hard of hearing, learning to use language is one of the highest of priorities. Language is best learned in interaction with others who know and use language. There is no substitute for reading along with another person and having a discussion of the reading, and so this human function cannot be turned over to a machine.

Once a child has learned to read some, I believe there is benefit to be gained by some use of computer games that require reading and writing in order to follow directions, because a close reading is necessary in order to do well in the game. Still, such activities cannot substitute for listening to and speaking with real people that is the foundation for authentic reading.

16. How do we get creative writing while ensuring proper grammatical text?

First, I think one must ask why and for what purposes "proper" usage is desirable. In some instances, conventional usage is not necessary. In others, it may not even be possible. For example, when a person is taking notes or brainstorming a list of possibilities, the ideas may be flying so fast that if he or she stopped to decide how to express them conventionally, they may be lost. Creativity demands being able to play with the language in order to discover and create new meanings. Putting too many demands at once on the overall process will get in the way of the writer saying much of anything that is satisfying or important. Sometimes just getting the beginnings down on paper is more important than being "proper" about it.

After the preliminary ideas are down on paper, though, the writer needs to read her or his language carefully and make the necessary corrections resulting in conventional usage. Otherwise, the writing will not communicate successfully. Children can be taught that writing involves going through a series of steps that aim progressively toward the development of their ideas expressed in clear and conventional language. Therefore, whether a particular piece of writing should be required to be "proper" or not depends on what stage of the writing process the piece represents. Brainstorming and preliminary drafts need not be required to be in conventional language; final drafts should exhibit conventional language use.

Because of continuous exposure to well-formed sentences and paragraphs, the child who is deaf or hard of hearing who reads frequently has a good chance of knowing well the conventions of good written language and will likely be in a good position to write in "proper" ways.

8

How Much Should Parents, Therapists, and Teachers Push?

Highlight

▼ Adults in the child's life should provide a loving, stimulating, and well-balanced language-rich environment in which the child can learn.

A PARENT ASKS WHETHER TO PUSH A $4^1/_2$-YEAR-OLD WHO ENJOYS MAKING "chicken scratches" to write "real" letters. Another asks if the 2-year-old needs to learn to read and write. Still another feels that children should be left alone to learn what interests them. Her child is 7 and shows no signs of beginning to read.

There are, obviously, many points of view parents take concerning their children's learning, whether they are thinking about reading and writing or any other area of life. Some parents see life as a competition and want their children to have every advantage so they can "get ahead." They want even their very young children to produce achievements that would make a school-aged child outstanding, believing this is insurance for getting ahead and staying ahead. At the other extreme, some parents take the view that "nature will take its course," believing there is not much they can do to influence their children's achievement. Both such extremes are found in parents who have children who are deaf or hard of hearing as well as children who have normal hearing. It's easy to look around and see both approaches, whether one is in the neighborhood elementary school or in the speech and language clinic.

Add to these extremes the fact that most parents receive little education on child development. Most do not know what to expect from their children or anyone else's children, whether they have normal hearing or not. Conversations among parents of small children often center around how early and how often each parent's child does this or that, with the parent whose child has not done something as early as another child feeling diminished, as though later walking or talking makes one inferior. "What — he doesn't know his letters yet? My Bobby could say them all when he was 2!" can strike terror into any parent. The alternative for some is to opt out of such competition and go for the other extreme of saying (and hoping) it will all somehow take care of itself.

I well remember these talks, the "one-upsmanship" involved, and the feelings surrounding them, and am very grateful to the wise person who said to me "You know, when Annie's 18, you'll probably never be asked when she started talking. The important thing is that she learn as much about talking as possible." This, to me, begins to define the middle ground between the two extremes. First, the statement identifies a goal, that of the child fulfilling her or his potential. Second, it accepts that potential, whatever it turns out to be. And third, rather than setting a timetable, it leaves room for expectations to change as the child changes.

But what is possible? It is important to have high expectations for the child, but high expectations are not license to badger the child, thinking that doing so will result in high achievement. Instead, high expectations for the child who is deaf or hard of hearing can come from knowing that many other children who are deaf or hard of hearing have achieved well. Knowing this, the parent's task is to become as informed as possible about the "normal" developmental milestones and the typical earliest and latest times at which they occur in most children. For example, the *average* child begins to walk alone at 11 months and 3 weeks, but the span within which 90% of children begin to walk alone is 9 to 17 months (Berk, 1994, p. 149). The ability to produce a two-word sentence emerges in children with normal hearing between $1\frac{1}{2}$ and $2\frac{1}{2}$ years, a fairly long span of time (Berk, 1994, p. 370). Some children begin very early; others much later. This is normal. Understanding the normal span of development for a particular achievement can help parents decide when to help the child with that skill, when to sit back and wait, and when to turn to an expert for help. Knowing about the span of development informs us that $4\frac{1}{2}$-year-olds can be very normal and not be writing "real" letters and that 2-year-olds should not be expected to know the alphabet, much less be able to do any meaningful reading and writing. It also informs us that as the child gets toward the end of the normal span without having developed a particular ability, that letting it go and just hoping for the best is probably unwise.

In responding to the question of whether to push the child who is deaf or hard of hearing, I would want first to know what is meant by "pushing." To me, "pushing" suggests some kind of unreasonable pressure on the child. On the other hand, taking the child who is deaf or hard of hearing to speech and language therapy and doing everything one can to establish an enriched language environment does not sound to me like "pushing." I do not think the parent of a child who is deaf or hard of hearing has any choice but to act to create such an environment. Perhaps the person the parent should be "pushing" is the parent her or himself. I know it is hard work from the parent's point of view to take the child to speech and language sessions and then to plan and carry out one's own formal and informal teaching sessions throughout the week. It's hard to learn how to make the most possible from every casual language exchange with the child. But it's necessary. To do otherwise is to shrink back from helping the child achieve according to his or her potential. From the child's point of view, the many, many sessions need to feel like play. If so, the child doesn't feel unnaturally "pushed" (even though the parent does!). We should be able to assume more maturity from the parent than from the child, after all.

The same goes for reading and writing. Making sure the child is read to daily, is encouraged to make some choices about the stories, and has access to many written materials and crayons, paper, and pencils constitutes providing a print-enriched environment for the child. Conversing with the child even though he or she may not be answering helps. Pointing out the letters and talking about their "sounds" as the child seems ready for them adds to that environment. All of these help the child develop literacy abilities. Making the child repeat letters after the adult says them or match letters on workbook pages is pushing. Encouraging the child to pay attention all the way through to the end of the book (even skipping over some pages if necessary) is helpful, but getting into a battle over control of the book or whether a story will be read or not is pushing.

The task of the adult is to help the child increase in self-confidence by providing a stimulating and interesting environment in which the child receives legitimate and positive responses most of the time. The adult's praise must be easy to get, but it must also be legitimate. Hearing "Good job, Jane!" when she knows she did not try very hard does not add to Jane's self-confidence; instead Jane learns that Mom doesn't have very high standards and neither should she. She also learns that she doesn't have to stretch herself at all for Mom. Good self-confidence comes in part from trying to do something one couldn't do before and succeeding at it. The wise adult looks at the child's achievement, gauges where learning might best occur next, and sets up the situation.

Parents, therapists, and teachers should not "push"; instead they should work together to nurture an increasingly complex progression of development in the particular child, always taking into account the child's interests, strengths, and emotional well-being. This is best accomplished by knowing the child well and by seeking to make a little bit of progress each day in language learning, reading, and writing.

Epilogue

MY EXPERIENCES GROWING UP WITH A SEVERE-TO-PROFOUND HEARING LOSS WERE positive. While I did have times where I felt life was unfair to me, they didn't last long, because my parents always told me I was special and took the time to talk to me about my feelings. They didn't single me out or treat me differently because of my hearing loss. They treated both my brother and me the same; he often participated in home therapy sessions with me. I was mainstreamed all my life in school and have now graduated from Kalamazoo College.

There were many different things I remember my parents doing with me at an early age to help me. One of my favorite things we did was to keep an "Experience Book" which was a journal where we would draw pictures illustrating what we had done that day with simple sentences and words describing the pictures. These books helped me learn how to read and fostered my love of reading. Knowing how to spell words and read was important for me; it was another form of communication for me and aided in my understanding of spoken words. The Experience Books also gave me an early start in journal writing, which I've kept from middle school to the present, as a way to express my feelings, thoughts, fears, and dreams.

I went to many different therapists when I was younger. The ones I remember the most were Helen Beebe and Mary Koch from the Helen Beebe Speech and Hearing Center in Pennsylvania, Deborah Baxter, and Barb Lechner. I remember Beebe's because we would go for a week each year and stay in the Larry Jarret House. It made therapy and learning fun for me at that impressionable young age. I learned the best in interactive environments where I was actively talking and sharing.

I was required to start speech therapy in kindergarten and all the way through fifth grade to improve my speech. I intensely disliked going to therapy, but my parents insisted that I keep going because it was good for me. When I entered sixth grade I decided on my own to stop going to the school speech therapist. My parents didn't force me to keep going; they let me make my own decision. I never went back to therapy on a regular basis after that. By the time I reached high school I realized what all the therapy was for. I was thankful I could talk as well as I do.

One thing people are always surprised to discover is that I can talk on the phone. It was really hard for me at first but with the help and encouragement of my parents, it eventually got a lot easier and now I'm able to hold conversations over the phone.

While most people may see many disadvantages to having a hearing loss, I can certainly counter them with the advantages. Several advantages, among many, include being able to concentrate really well and stay focused on activities for long periods of time; being able to turn off my hearing aids if things are too loud or if I don't want to listen to anyone; and being able to read other people's body language very well, making me a very intuitive and sensitive person to other people's needs and feelings.

There is no doubt that it has taken a lot of work and patience from many people to help me get to the point where I am today. Right now I am eagerly looking forward to starting my new full-time job as an admission counselor at my alma mater. I will be traveling to meet with prospective students and their families, attending college fairs and admission counselor conferences, and representing the College. I feel that I can set out to accomplish anything I set my mind to. I would not be the person I am today if it were not for the patience and stamina of my parents, the guidance of my therapists, and the feelings instilled within me that I am worth a whole lot and can achieve many things in my lifetime.

Annie Robertson
June 2000

References

Adams, M.J. (1991). *Beginning to read.* Cambridge, MA: The MIT Press.

The American Heritage Dictionary (1985). Boston: Houghton Mifflin Company.

Anderson, R.C., & Pearson, P.D. (1984). A schema-theoretic view of basic processes in reading comprehension. In P.D. Pearson (Ed.), *Handbook of Reading Research* (pp. 255-292). New York: Longman.

Allen, T.E. (1986). Patterns of academic achievement among hearing impaired students: 1974 and 1983. In A.N. Schildroth & M.A. Karchmer (Eds.), *Deaf children in America* (pp. 161-206). San Diego, CA: College-Hill Press.

Altwerger, B., Edelsky, C., & Flores, B. (1987). Whole language: What's new? *The Reading Teacher, 41,* 144-154.

Ashton-Warner, S. (1963, 1986). *Teacher.* New York: Simon and Schuster.

Auditory-Verbal International (1991). Auditory-verbal position statement. *The Auricle, 4,* 11-12.

Austen, J. (1811, Reprinted 1992). *Sense and sensibility.* Denmark: Wordsworth Editions Limited.

Baron, N.S. (1995). Rembrandt at the sixteenth chapel: Demystifying language acquisition. In C.N. Hedley, P. Antonacci, & M. Rabinowitz (Eds.), *Thinking and literacy: The mind at work* (pp. 127-140). Hillsdale, NJ: Lawrence Erlbaum Associates.

Barron, R.W. (1987). Word recognition in early reading: A review of the direct and indirect access hypotheses. In P. Bertelson (Ed.), *The onset of literacy.* Cambridge, MA: MIT Press.

Beebe, H.H. (1976). Deaf children can learn to hear. In G.W. Nix (Ed.), *Mainstream education of hearing impaired children and youth.* Philadelphia: Grune & Stratton.

Berk, L. (1994). *Child development.* Boston: Allyn and Bacon.

Bernhardt, R., & Antonacci, P. (1995). In search of thinking environments. In C.N. Hedley, P. Antonacci, & M. Rabinowitz (Eds.), *Thinking and literacy: The mind at work* (pp. 241-255). Hillsdale, NJ: Lawrence Erlbaum Associates.

Bloom, B.S. (1956). *Taxonomy of educational objectives: Handbook I — Cognitive domain.* New York: Longman, Green, and Co.

Britton, J. (1993). *Language and learning.* Portsmouth, NH: Boynton Cook.

Clay, M. (1990). Concepts about print in English and other languages. *The Reading Teacher, 42,* 268-276.

Cleary, B. (1968). *Ramona the Pest.* New York: William Morrow and Company.

Clifford, C. (1989). Man/woman/teacher: Gender, family, and career in American educational history. In D. Warren (Ed.), *American teachers: Histories of a profession at work.* New York: Macmillan, pp. 307-308.

Duffy, G.G., & G.B. Sherman. (1972). *Systematic reading instruction.* New York: Harper and Row.

Durkin, D. (1966). *Children who read early.* New York: Teachers College Press.

Durkin, D. (1993). *Teaching them to read* (6th ed.). Boston: Allyn and Bacon.

Ehri, L. (1995). Teachers need to know how word reading processes develop to teach reading effectively to beginners. In C.N. Hedley, P. Antonacci, & M. Rabinowitz (Eds.), *Thinking and literacy: The mind at work* (pp. 167-188). Hillsdale, NJ: Lawrence Erlbaum Associates.

Estabrooks, W. (1994). *Auditory-verbal therapy for parents and professionals.* Washington, DC: Alexander Graham Bell Association for the Deaf and Hard of Hearing.

Ferreiro, E. (1991). Literacy acquisition and the representation of language. In C. Kamii, M. Manning, & G. Manning (Eds.), *Early literacy: A constructivist foundation for whole language.* Washington, DC: National Education Association.

Ferreiro, E. (1990). Literacy development: Psychogenesis. In Y.M. Goodman (Ed.), *How children construct literacy.* Newark, DE: International Reading Association.

Flexer, C. (1994). *Facilitating hearing and listening in young children.* San Diego, CA: Singular Publishing Company.

Fry, D.B. (1966). The development of the phonological system in the normal and the deaf child. In F. Smith & G.A. Miller (Eds.), *The genesis of language: A psycholinguistic approach* (pp. 187-206). Cambridge, MA: The MIT Press.

Geers, A.S., & Moog, J.S. (1989). Factors predictive of the development of literacy in profoundly hearing-impaired adolescents. *The Volta Review, 91,* 69-86.

Goldberg, D. (Ed.). (1993). Auditory-verbal philosophy: A tutorial. *The Volta Review, 95,* 181-263.

Goldberg, D., & Flexer, C. (1993). Outcome survey of auditory-verbal graduates — Study of clinical efficacy. *Journal of the American Academy of Audiology, 4,* 189-200.

Goodman, Y. (1990). Children's knowledge about literacy development: An afterword. In Y.M. Goodman (Ed.), *How children construct literacy.* Newark, DE: International Reading Association.

Griffith, P., & Olson, M. (1992). Phonemic awareness helps beginning readers break the code. *The Reading Teacher, 45*(7), 516-523.

Grossi, E. (1990). Applying psychogenesis principles to the literacy instruction of lower-class children in Brazil. In Y.M. Goodman (Ed.), *How children construct literacy.* Newark, DE: International Reading Association.

Hansen, J., & Graves, D. (1992). Unifying the English language arts curriculum. In J. Flood, J.M. Jensen, D. Lapp, & J.R. Squire (Eds.), *Handbook of research on teaching the English language arts* (pp. 805-819). New York: Macmillan.

Hart, B. (1978). *Teaching reading to deaf children.* Jackson Heights, NY: Lexington School for the Deaf.

Heath, S.B. (1994). The children of Trackton's children: Spoken and written language in social change. In R.B. Ruddell, M.R. Ruddell, & H. Singer (Eds.), *Theoretical models and processes of reading.* Newark, DE: International Reading Association, pp. 208-230.

Hedley, C., & Hedley, W. (1995). Thinking and literary: The mind at work in the classroom. In C.N. Hedley, P. Antonacci, & M. Rabinowitz (Eds.), *Thinking and literacy: The mind at work* (pp. 3-20). Hillsdale, NJ: Lawrence Erlbaum Associates.

Juell, C., Griffith, P.L., & Gough, P.B. (1986). Acquisition of literacy: A longitudinal study of children in first and second grade. *Journal of Educational Psychology, 78,* 243-255.

Kamii, C., Manning, M., & Manning, G. (1991). *Early literacy: A constructivist foundation for whole language.* Washington, DC: National Education Association.

Kamii, C. (1991). What is constructivism? In C. Kamii, M. Manning, & G. Manning (Eds.), *Early literacy: A constructivist foundation for whole language* (pp. 17-30). Washington, DC: National Education Association.

King, C., & Quigley, S. (1985). *Reading and deafness.* San Diego, CA: College-Hill Press.

Kozol, J. (1985). *Illiterate America.* New York: New American Library.

Lane, H., & Baker, D. (1974). Reading achievement of the deaf: Another look. *The Volta Review, 76,* 488-499.

Lefrancois, G. (1991). *Psychology for Teaching.* Belmont, CA: Wadsworth Publishing Company.

Lewis, B.S., & Long, R. (1991). Reading to know. In C. Kamii, M. Manning, & G. Manning (Eds.), *Early literacy: A constructivist foundation for whole language* (pp. 119-128). Washington, DC: National Education Association.

Ling, D. (1993). Auditory-verbal options for children with hearing impairment: Helping to pioneer and applied science. *The Volta Review, 95,* 187-196.

Ling, D. (1989). *Foundations of spoken language for hearing-impaired children.* Washington, DC: Alexander Graham Bell Association for the Deaf and Hard of Hearing.

Ling, A. (1977). *Schedules of development in audition, speech, language, and communication for hearing impaired infants and their families.* Washington, DC: Alexander Graham Bell Association for the Deaf and Hard of Hearing.

Ling, D., & Ling, A. (1978). *Aural habilitation: The foundations of verbal learning in hearing-impaired children.* Washington, DC: Alexander Graham Bell Association for the Deaf and Hard of Hearing.

Lou, M.W. (1988). The history of language use in the education of the Deaf in the United States. In M. Strong (Ed.), *Language learning and deafness* (pp. 75-98). Cambridge, U.K.: Cambridge University Press.

Lyons, C., Pinnell, G., & DeFord, D., (1993). *Partners in learning: Teachers and children in reading recovery.* New York: Teachers College Press.

Marzano, R. (1995). Enhancing thinking and reasoning in the English language arts. In C.N. Hedley, P. Antonacci, & M. Rabinowitz (Eds.), *Thinking and literacy: The mind at work* (pp. 73-100). Hillsdale, NJ: Lawrence Erlbaum Associates.

Meadow, K.P. (1980). *Deafness and child development.* Berkeley: University of California Press.

Moog, J.S., & Geers, A.S. (1985). EPIC: A Program to accelerate academic progress in profoundly hearing-impaired children. *The Volta Review, 87,* 259-277.

Pauk, W. (1989). *How to Study in College.* Boston: Houghton Mifflin.

Pearson, P.D., & Stephens, D. (1994). Learning about literacy: A 30-year journey. In R.B. Ruddell, M.R. Ruddell, & H. Singer (Eds.), *Theoretical models and processes of reading.* (pp. 22-42). Newark, DE: International Reading Association.

Pintner, R., & Patterson, D.G. (1916). Learning tests with deaf children. *Psychology Monographs, 20.*

Pollack, D. (1985). *Educational audiology for the limited-hearing infant and preschooler* (2nd ed.). Springfield, IL: Charles C. Thomas.

Pollack, D. (1993). Reflections of a pioneer. *The Volta Review, 95,* 197-204.

Robertson, L. (under review). *Reading and writing achievement of children with hearing impairment taught through the auditory-verbal approach.*

Robertson, L., & Flexer, C. (1993). Reading development: A survey of children with hearing loss who developed speech and language through the auditory-verbal method. *The Volta Review, 95,* 253-261.

Ruddell, R.B., & Ruddell, M.R. (1994). Language acquisition and literacy processes. In R.B. Ruddell, M.R. Ruddell, & H. Singer (Eds.), *Theoretical models and processes of reading.* Newark, DE: International Reading Association, pp. 83-103.

Rumelhart, D.E. (1985). Toward an interactive model of reading. In Singer, H., & Ruddell (Eds.), *Theoretical models and processes of reading.* Newark, DE: International Reading Association.

Rumelhart, D.E. (1977). The representation of knowledge in memory. In R.C. Anderson & R.J. Spiro (Eds.), *Schooling and the acquisition of knowledge.* Hillsdale, NJ: Lawrence Erlbaum Associates.

Samuels, S. J. (1994). Word recognition. In R.B. Ruddell, M.R. Ruddell, & H. Singer (Eds.), *Theoretical models and processes of reading.* Newark, DE: International Reading Association, pp. 359-380.

Schildroth, A.N., & Karchmer, M.A. (Eds.) (1986). *Deaf children in America.* San Diego, CA: College-Hill Press.

Schlesinger, H. (1988). Questions and answers in the development of deaf children. In M. Strong (Ed.), *Language learning and deafness* (pp. 261-291). Cambridge, U.K.: Cambridge University Press.

Dr. Seuss (1993). *The cat in the hat.* Westminster, MD: Random Books Young Reader.

Shannon, P. (1989). *Broken promises: Reading instruction in twentieth century America.* New York: Bergin and Garvey.

Smith, F. (1985). *Reading without nonsense.* New York: Teachers College Press.

Smith, F. (1978). *Understanding reading: A psycholinguistic analysis of reading and learning to read* (2nd ed.) Newark, DE: International Reading Association.

Smith, F. (1982). *Writing and the writer.* New York: Holt, Rinehart and Winston.

Stokoe, W.C. (1960). Sign language structure: An outline of the visual communication systems of the American deaf. *Studies in Linguistics, 8.*

Teale, W.H. (1978). Positive environments for learning to read: What studies of early readers tell us. *Language Arts, 55,* 922-932.

Teale, W.H. (1981). Parents reading to their children: What we know and what we need to know. *Language Arts, 58,* 902-912.

Vaughan, P. (Ed.) (1976). *Learning to listen: A book by mothers for mothers of hearing-impaired children.* Don Mills, Ontario, Canada: New Press.

Vygotsky, L. (1962). *Thought and language.* Cambridge, MA: The MIT Press.

Walser, N. (1998). Learning to listen may help children learn to read. *The Harvard Education Letter, 14*(6), 1-4.

Wedenberg, E. (1951). *Auditory training for deaf and hard of hearing children.* Stockholm: Victor Pettersons Bokindustriaktiebolag.

Appendix I: Holistic Scale for Evaluating Writing, K–12

Level 4 ____Topic is carefully organized with appropriate supporting details.
____Good vocabulary and varied word choices for grade level.
____Purpose is focused on audience/reader.
____Good sentence structure, showing variety and style.
____Very few errors in MUGS (Mechanics, Usage, Grammar, Spelling).
____Shows creativity and originality.

Level 3 ____Topic is developed with some supporting details.
____Appropriate vocabulary and word choice for grade level.
____Some awareness of audience/reader.
____Some varied sentence structure with few fragments or run-ons.
____Some problems with MUGS.
____Shows some creativity in addressing the topic.

Level 2 ____Strays from topic with few supporting details.
____Limited vocabulary and word choice for grade level.
____Limited awareness of audience/reader.
____Basic sentence structure with limited variety and some sentence fragments or run-ons.
____MUGS begin to interfere with meaning.
____Shows limited creativity in addressing the topic.

Level 1 ____Topic is poorly developed.
____Simple vocabulary and poor word choice for grade level.

____No sense of audience/reader.
____Contains limited sentence structures and many sentence fragments or run-ons.
____Major problems with MUGS.
____Shows no creativity in addressing the topic.

Appendix II: Favorite Books for Different Ages

MANY LISTS HAVE BEEN CREATED OF OUTSTANDING BOOKS FOR CHILDREN, AND your public library and the Internet are good sources for these lists. Each year, the American Library Association gives three awards for books its panels judge to be outstanding:

- ▼ The Newbery Medal (the best American children's book of the year)
    http://www.ala.org/alsc/newbery.html

- ▼ The Caldecott Medal (best picture book of the year)
    http://www.ala.org/alsc/caldecott.html

- ▼ Notable Children's Books
    http://www.ala.org/alsc/nbook99.html

Favorite Books

I also like asking librarians and teachers for their own favorites, because they have seen how children react to them. Here is a list given to me recently by Lesley Torello (children's librarian of the Granville Public Library, Granville, Ohio), JanaVon Dach, Noreen Pinkerton, Sherri McCaul, Diana Jones, Mary Ann Yanes, Kristine Michael, and Barbara Klatt (teachers at Granville Elementary School, Granville, Ohio).

PRESCHOOL
Charlie Needs a Cloak (T. DePaola)
Miss Spider's Tea Party (D. Kirk)
The Outside Inn (G. Lyon)
Too Much Noise (A. McGovern)
The Glerp (D. McPhail)
Mouse TV (M. Novak)
Mother, Mother I Want Another (M. Polushkin)

Any Kind of Dog (L. Reiser)
Caps for Sale (E. Slobodkina)
Yoko (R. Wells)

KINDERGARTEN
The Polar Express (C. Van Allsburg)
Ira Sleeps Over (B. Waber)
The Animal (L. Balian)
Love You, Forever (R. Munsch)
Swimmy (L. Lionni)
The Rainbow Fish (M. Pfister)
Is Your Mama a Llama? (D. Guarino)
Children of the Earth — Remember (S. Schimmel)
Chicka Chicka Boom Boomx (B. Martin)
Chrysanthemum (K. Henkes)

FIRST GRADE
Strega Nona (T. Depaola)
James and the Giant Peach (R. Dahl)
Owl Moon (J. Yolen)
Officer Buckle and Gloria (P. Rathmann)
If You Give a Mouse a Cookie (L. Numeroff)
A House for Hermit Crab (E. Carle)
Miss Rumphins (B. Cooney)
Sylvester and the Magic Pebble (W. Steig)
Where the Wild Things Are (M. Sendak)
Frog and Toad (series) (A. Lobel)

SECOND GRADE
Tops and Bottoms (J. Stevens)
Amelia Bedelia (P. Parish)
Arthur Babysits (M. Brown)
Thundercake (P. Polarco)
The Empty Pot (Demi)
The King's Commissioners (A. Friedman)
A Cloak for a Dreamer (A. Friedman)
Abe Lincoln's Hat (M. Brenner)
A Pizza the Size of the Sun (J. Prelutsky)
Encyclopedia Brown (series) (D. Sobol)

THIRD GRADE
Sarah, Plain and Tall (P. McLachlan)
Charlotte's Web (E.B. White)
The Boxcar Children (series) (G.C. Warner)
The Secret Garden (F.H. Burnett)

Indian in the Cupboard (L.R. Banks)
Mr. Popper's Penguins (R. Atwater)
Castle in the Attic (E. Winthrop)
The BFG (R. Dahl)
What's the Big Idea, Ben Franklin? (J. Fritz)
How To Be Cool in the Third Grade (B. Duffey)

FOURTH GRADE
Shiloh (P. Naylor)
Danny, Champion of the World (R. Dahl)
Anastasia Krupnik (L. Lowry)
Harry Potter and the Sorceror's Stone (J. Rowling)
The Kid in the Red Jacket (B. Park)
Superfudge (J. Blume)
Bunnicula (D. Howe)
Ella Enchanted (G. Levine)
The Music of Dolphins (K. Hesse)
Hatchet (G. Paulsen)

FIFTH GRADE
The Not-Just-Anybody Family (B. Byars)
Two Against the Tide (B. Clements)
A Wrinkle in Time (M. L'Engle)
George Washington's Socks (E. Woodruff)
Shh! They're Writing the Constitution (J. Fritz)
Bonanza Girl (P. Beatty)
Shades of Gray (C. Reeder)
In the Year of the Boar and Jackie Robinson (B. Lord)
Hello, My Name is Scramble Eggs (J. Gilson)
To Walk the Sky Path (P. Naylor)

Appendix III: Auditory-Verbal Centers

(All have Certified Auditory-Verbal Therapists [Cert. AVT] on staff.)

Auditory-Verbal International, Inc. (AVI)
2121 Eisenhower Avenue
Suite 402
Alexandria, VA 22314
(703) 739-1049
audiverb@aol.com
(call for a list of Certified Auditory-Verbal Therapists, or visit the AVI website)

UNITED STATES

Auditory-Verbal Center of Atlanta, Inc.
Maggy Harms, Executive Director
1447 Peachtree Street, Suite 210
Atlanta, GA 30309
(404) 815-4321
www.avc-atlanta@mindspring.com

Auditory-Verbal Communication Center
James Watson
544 Washington Street
Gloucester, MA 01930
(508) 282-0025

The Bolesta Center
Chellie Lisenby, Executive Director
7205 N. Habana Avenue
Tampa, FL 33614
(813) 932-1184
fax (813) 932-9583
www.bolesta.com

Chattering Children
Pratibha Srinivasan, Executive Director
9507 Hill Street Road
Suite C1
Richmond, VA 23236
(804) 745-0915
fax (804) 745-2734
www.chatchild@mindspring.com

Educational Audiology Programs
Marian Ernst, Director
1077 South Gilpin Street
Denver, CO 80209
(303) 777-0740

Flower Hospital
T.A.L.K. Program
Linda Wood-Gottfried
5100 Harroun Road
Sylvania, OH 43560
(419) 824-1067
fax (419) 824-1773
rlgottfried@toast.net

Helen Beebe Speech and Hearing Center
Amanda Mangiardi, Executive Director
220 Commerce Drive, Suite 320
Fort Washington, PA 19034
(215) 619-9083
fax (215) 619-9087
www.beebecen@netaxs.com

Listen and Talk
George Olsen, Executive Director
20302 Bothell Way, NE
Bothell, WA 98011
(425) 483-9700
www.hear@listentalk.org

Listen Foundation
Sheri Clark, Executive Director
300 E. Hampton, Suite 304
Englewood, CO 80110-2659
(303) 781-9440
(303) 781-2018
www.lstnfoun@aol.com

Phoenix Center
Victoria Deasy, Executive Director
1291 East Hillsdale Boulevard
Suite 123
Foster City, CA 94404
(650) 570-6369
fax (650) 570-6367

Talk Center
Linda Daniels, Executive Director
P.O. Box 670805
Dallas, TX 75367-0805
(214) 373-4357

The University of Akron
Denise Wray, Director of AVT Program
Audiology and Speech Center
The University of Akron
Akron, OH 44325-3001
(330) 972-8188
fax (330) 972-7884

University of South Carolina
Speech and Hearing Center
Todd Houston, Director of A-V Program
1601 St. Julian Place
Columbia, SC 29204
(803) 777-2614
fax (803) 738-4222
thouston@sc.edu

AUSTRALIA

The Hear and Say Centre for Deaf Children
Dimity Dornan, Director
40-44 Munro Street
Auchenflower, OLD
4066 Australia
011-67-7-3300-3401
fax 011-61-7-3870-3998
www.hearsay@powerup.com.au

CANADA

Auditory-Verbal Therapy Program
North York General Hospital
Warren Estabrooks, Director
10 Buchan Court
Toronto, Ontario M2J 1V4
Canada
(416) 491-4648
westabro@nygh.on.ca

Children's Hospital of Eastern Ontario
Elizabeth Fitzpatrick, Director
Audiology Department
401 Smyth Road
Ottawa, Ontario K1H 8L1
Canada
(613) 737-2378
fitzpatrick@cheo.on.ca

TAIWAN

The Children's Hearing Foundation
Judy Simser, Director
3F 128 Yu Ming Sixth Road
Taipei, Taiwan
02-2827-4550
fax 02-2827-4555
raysimoo@ms9.hinet.net

Index

ABOUT THE AUTHORS

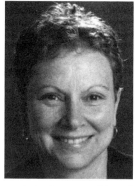

LYN ROBERTSON, PH.D.
DENISON UNIVERSITY, GRANVILLE, OH

Lyn Robertson is Associate Professor and Chair of the Department of Education at Denison University, a liberal arts college in Granville, Ohio. She holds a B.A. from Denison in English, an M.A. from Northwestern University in Reading and Language, and a Ph.D. from The Ohio State University in Reading with an emphasis on cognition. She taught students English and reading at the junior and senior high levels before moving to Denison, where she teaches and participates in all phases of teacher preparation. One strand of her research has centered on literacy and deafness, a subject dear to her heart. She is the mother of a now-grown child, a recent college graduate, who had a prelingual severe-to-profound hearing loss until receiving a cochlear implant in 1999 at the age of 21. This is her first book.

CAROL FLEXER, PH.D., PROFESSOR OF AUDIOLOGY
THE UNIVERSITY OF AKRON, AKRON, OHIO

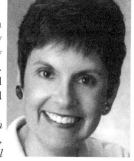

Carol Flexer received her doctorate in audiology from Kent State University in 1982. She has been at the University of Akron for 20 years, where she is a Professor of Audiology in the School of Speech-Language Pathology and Audiology. Special areas of expertise include pediatric and educational audiology. She has lectured internationally and authored more than 80 publications.

She has co-edited three books: *How the Student with Hearing Loss Can Succeed in College,* first and second editions, and *Sound-Field FM Amplification: Theory and Practical Applications.* She has authored fourth and fifth books titled, *Facilitating Hearing and Listening in Young Children* — first and second editions. The second edition was just published in 1999.

She is a past president of the Educational Audiology Association, a past Board member of Auditory-Verbal International, and a past president of the American Academy of Audiology.